To April,

A  boomers ROCK™ Book

Foreword by Todd Durkin, author of *The IMPACT! Body Plan*

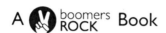
D1500742

Maximize Your Quality of Life

The 200% Solution

Tom Matt, BA/MA, CPT, FNS, NASM

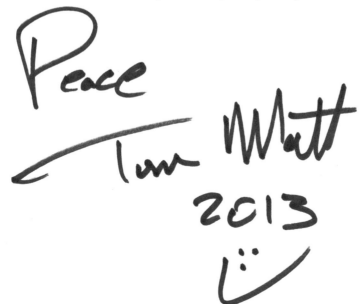

Peace

Tom Matt

2013

Maximize Your Quality of Life, The 200% Solution

Published by Boomers Rock, LLC
2231 Beechnut Trail
Holt, Michigan 48842
www.boomersrock.us

ISBN 978-0-9855470-0-4

Library of Congress number

1st Edition

Date of publication: August 2012

Cover and layout design by Kerrie Lian, under contract with MacGraphics Services (www.macgraphics.net).

Edited by Stephanie Pierce and Mickey Hadick.

Other publishing services provided by Hadick Enterprises, LLC.

"Walk No Beaches Barefoot" Copyright (C) 1986 by Brian Wallace. Used with his permission.

Disclaimers
The health and fitness information contained in this book should not be followed without first consulting your health care professional.

The information contained in this book is based on sources the author believes to be reliable.

Neither the author nor the publisher is responsible for websites or other sources cited that are not owned by the author or the publisher.

Please visit www.boomersrock.us for errata and new editions.

Walk No Beaches Barefoot

South Pacific charm
Femur of black moon
Some far-off land allows
An H-bomb blast
Round the world
I in the womb feel
The mantle bend to breathe

~Brian Wallace

Acknowledgements

In every aspect of my life I have been blessed to have many people who have supported, guided, listened and encouraged me to move forward and accomplish my journey of life. There is no doubt that without their help, kindness and understanding I would not be where I am today. Life is about finding mentors and building trust, loving your family, friends and never giving up.

I would first like to thank my wife Sandy for her patience and devotion. She tolerates and continues to give to me the direction and steadiness that I need to be successful. Without her there is no "Boomers Rock".

Next I have to thank Michigan State University and the College of Communication Arts and Sciences. The entire staff and faculty are among the many individuals who made the nine years of undergraduate and graduate work possible and achievable. Specifically, though, I would be remiss if I did not thank several individuals whose kindness, care, mentoring and guidance made my journey possible. Dr. Roy Simon was the very first of my mentors who gave me his time when the day was darkest at the very beginning of my academic quest. Without his support, college and growth would never have happened. Professor Johannes Bauer, my graduate advisor and friend who took me under his wing and gave me his time. Rachel Iseler, who became my friend and ersatz advisor through the whole college process and was incredibly kind. Professors Constantinos Coursaris, Steve Wildman, Kurt DeMaagd are just a few of the educators who instilled the skills I needed to be successful. Dean Pamela Whitten who has built a great team of educators through the entire college and been available and approachable at any turn, she has been great. And of course my main man, the late Professor Tom Muth, one of the key educators to ever enter my life and the lives of hundreds of other students. His loss was a soul never to be replaced, he truly was special. There are many more people who touched my life in the academic environment, suffice to say all are in my gratitude for their good will and support, thank you.

Mickey Hadick is my friend, partner and guidance counselor. Along with his belief in my quirkiness he saw something that needed to be channeled—my energy. He believed in the potential; when someone like Mickey helps you achieve lofty ambitions and goals you have a true diamond. Without his focus and advice, our ride into the stratosphere of life would not take place.

Regie Reider and Chris Johnson are friends who believed in me and through their kindness helped my journey; they will always be of paramount importance to me. Chris always saw my "juice", even when I had no idea what he was talking about. And Regie is my bro.

I want to thank Shawn Webb and Ermal Turkesi, the dynamic duo behind FTNS, the first all-fitness radio network. Shawn heard my story in the beginning and he is the one who saw something that is now becoming more than I could have ever dreamed. Without that first conversation one snowy February day, "Boomers Rock" never happens.

Phillipa Burgess and Dr. Ray Faulkenberry are two key individuals who became my friends and advisors. Without these two individuals, the rocket never leaves the pad. Without Ray's advice on making my list, and believing in myself, and without Phillipa's advice on writing the book, I am virtually clueless on my direction. Mentors and advisors can come from anywhere, at any time.

Motion Marketing, my man Pete Ruffing, Tiffany Dowling, Anna Daugherty,

Kelly Mazurkiewicz, and Mary McElgunn, who believed in my energy and passion and helped define the brand. Pete: just remember the hand with six fingers!

My gym pals, Nick Tijerina, Tom Mitchell, Vennie Gore, Patty Oehmke, Denise Rabi, and all of my other faculty friends who inspire me to keep on keeping on. All of the numerous students who I have worked with, worked out with, and become friends with, I hope they all realize how much it means to me to draw from their friendships and energy. It gives me the confidence to suggest to all baby boomers to build relationships with our younger people, mentoring and being mentored by our next generations. Vennie, thanks for turning me on to Malcolm Gladwell and his excellent books; you gave me advice, and I am forever thankful.

And David DeMarco, a real pro who has helped me understand the talk show business, the importance of reading daily, and that spiritual guidance and helping others is a talent and a gift.

Foreword

By Todd Durkin

I was first introduced to Tom Matt as a guest on his radio show, *Boomers Rock*, in August of 2011. As a strength and conditioning coach and personal trainer to dozens of elite and professional athletes in the NFL, NBA, and MLB, I was on the show to discuss how I work with my clients to help them become their best. To make them champions. World champions.

And I remember thinking to myself during the show, "Man, this Tom Matt guy has some serious world-class energy and passion himself. I LIKE THAT!"

And so it began. A relationship of mutual respect for the path and journey to help build world-class in others. For me, I have a "Train the Joes like the pros" mentality that allows me to train my thousands of male and female clients just like my elite athletes. And that includes hundreds of baby-boomers. For Tom, his sole focus is the baby-boomer. The interesting thing is that the characteristics for training pros and training boomers are amazingly similar.

The 200% Solution is a way of life. It's a culmination of Tom's wisdom and insights as a baby-boomer himself. It beautifully articulates history, knowledge, science, and personal experience.

Most importantly, this book will positively IMPACT you to take action and to build YOUR best life, regardless of age, background, circumstance, or experience. Tom Matt is an example of how you can overcome obstacle and challenge and thrive in life. But YOU must be willing to step up to The 200% Solution level.

I shared earlier that much of what Tom delivers in his book is similar to the messaging I share everyday in the trenches with my athletes and clients.

Get Your Mind Right. Tom eloquently and authentically talks about attitude and belief. This is huge. I believe it is imperative at ANY age, young or old, to make sure your mind stays positive and you remain an optimist. Tom shares his strategies and methods to help you 'keep your mind right' and this alone, is worth its weight in gold.

Play with passion. Energy. "Nothing great in life was ever done without enthusiasm," says Ralph Waldo Emerson. I always tell my athletes to play with passion. It's the only way to play the game. And I believe we are either 'energy givers' or 'energy suckers'. I tell my clients not to be energy suckers. Give energy and give some more. And make sure it's positive. Maybe your game is tennis... or golf... or softball... or fitness... or maybe just life. Bottom line is this: Play All Out. Play with PASSION, play with enthusiasm, and play to "win."

Be willing to change and adapt. Wow, this is a big one. There are so many sayings about "change":

"Change or die."

"You choose change… or change will choose you."

"Embrace change."

Easier said then done, correct? I get it. But when Tom steps you back through time and you reminisce about the 1960s, 70s, 80s on up, you can see how much we really have changed as a country and as a culture.

Furthermore, he passionately talks about what we must CHANGE TODAY to guide our habits, mindset, attitude, and physical health. Reading The 200% Solution, I felt like I was 25 years younger, back in the locker room, and ready to PLAY again.

We all need a good kick in the backside every now and then. Tom Matt's pearls of wisdom provide the necessary steps to create positive change in life.

"You can't out-train a bad diet." I have been reciting this saying to my athletes and clients for years. As a fitness professional with 20+ years of experience, I can tell you that exercise and training will only get you so far if you eat don't right.

If you want radiant energy and vibrant health, you MUST eat right.

If you want to think clearly and keep mental focus and clarity, you must eat right.

If you want to change your body composition and decrease fat, you must eat right.

If you want to stave off arthritis, heart disease, and Type-II diabetes, boost your immunity, and even protect against certain forms of cancer, you must eat right.

If you want to LIVE, you must eat right.

The 200% Solution provides a world-class eating program for you to follow. It's simple—FOLLOW IT!

Physical conditioning is the foundation to drive success in all areas of your life. And yes, as a boomer, it's even more important that you get STRONG and stay STRONG.

Lift weights. It's essential for bone density and will keep you functionally strong.

Do cardio. I always say, "More cardio... less lardio." Just be smart. Maybe you can't run on the pavement like you used to. But you can swim, play tennis, or hop on a cardio piece like an elliptical, treadmill, or bike. You just have to have the discipline, consistency and commitment to make it part of your lifestyle.

The 200% Solution does a GREAT job providing you all you need to get fit and stay fit. And I know that if you follow Tom's program, you will be stronger, your energy will be more vibrant, and your life will be better. 200% better!

Never let age get in your way. Tom Matt and The 200% Solution will help you carve out your best life. By including his program as part of your everyday life, I know you will be grateful for Tom's words and insight.

As I have told Tom before, "Everyone has a LIFE worth telling a story about." The 200% Solution WILL help you create your best version of YOU. Your best years are ahead of you and I encourage you to continue to play with passion, live with purpose, and create IMPACT everyday.

Much love.

Todd Durkin, MA, CSCS
Owner, Fitness Quest 10 (San Diego, CA)
Author, *The IMPACT! Body Plan*
www.ToddDurkin.com

Dedication

To Sandy, Ashley Ann, Matt and LoLo: my love for all of you is my driving force. This book is dedicated to you all.

Table of Contents

Preface

I had to drop out of college to appreciate education.

I had to endure a failed marriage to appreciate love.

I had to live through alcohol and drug use to appreciate a clear mind.

I had to nearly die to appreciate my life.

I finally became accountable for my own actions, admitted to myself that I had not fulfilled my dreams, and became a better person.

Your moment could be anything: an illness, a loss, an accident, or a dream. It is what you do and how you act and react to your moment—*your epiphany*. This is your decision, the compelling 'how'. This book will help you toward a path of change and improvement.

This book can help you improve your quality of life. For a given person, improved physical fitness may be the key to their improved quality of life. For someone else, it might be motivation to embark on a new career or achieve a lifelong dream. For others still, it might be finding the combination of nutritional changes that provides the energy which makes a difference in their afternoon or evenings leading to new-found pleasures.

Some Boomers may be facing the modern era with a nostalgia that limits their experiences, and leads to regrets for missed opportunities in their life. This book is intended to help you face the future with a renewed vigor. Success in life often demands bold action, and we all may be challenged to summon the necessary courage. The 200% Solution is a synthesis of improved thinking patterns, nutritional strategies, and physical movements that lead to improved quality of life. The 200% Solution will maximize your quality of life.

If, after reading this book and employing the recommended techniques, you don't see marked improvements in your quality of life, then we will refund the cost of this book.

That's right—The 200% Solution comes with a 100% guarantee.

Now is the time to give yourself the best chance to enjoy the rest of your life.

Now is the time for The 200% Solution.

Part 0:

I AM BORN

I was born, just like seventy-nine million other Americans, in what was known as the "Baby Boom," bred by what was later called "The Greatest Generation." We grew up under the threat of nuclear annihilation while stuffing ourselves with Wonder Bread and Twinkies. Did our parents really think we were going to turn out just like they did?

We won the Cold War, survived the Vietnam War, settled some weird politics and then rode an economic roller coaster into what was supposed to be our golden years, the pot of gold at the end of the rainbow of our careers.

The world has a funny way of doing things the way it wants to, and has dealt our country a fresh set of geopolitical problems, just as your body has a funny way of becoming nothing like you thought it would, and it may seem that the best you can hope for is that you keep your wits about you while you watch old movies streamed to a digital television.

Or maybe the best you can hope for is to forget how good it felt to be young.

Facing your golden years does not have to be dreadful. I have discovered an approach to life, every aspect of life, that improved my quality of life. It can improve the quality of yours, too. I call it "The 200% Solution."

Coaches have urged their players to give 110% when competing if they wanted to win. That's not enough. We need to give 200%.

The best part is that giving 200% isn't any more difficult than giving 100%, and it will make you feel so good about life that you may want to give more. You won't have to, though. The 200% Solution will double the quality of your life. I guarantee it.

1: Introduction

My epiphany was an unplanned moment with my pulmonologist following a very severe and sudden illness. Bi-lateral pneumonia, possible tuberculosis, two days in the isolation ward of the hospital (where they wear the spacesuits to come in and treat you), six days total in the hospital.

I asked the doctor during my post-recovery visit two weeks later "How did this happen?" and, "Why me?"

The doctor replied matter-of-factly, "You probably carried this condition around for a long time, and it's only because you were in pretty good shape physically that you recovered." This was interesting, I thought. "Many people take months to recover from such a severe case like yours, and some don't even make it."

At that moment I knew in my heart that I had a decision to make, and I never wanted to go through this again. I was too young to become decrepit in a heartbeat.

It was at that point that I realized I had become a better person.

Epiphany, lightning, or divine intervention; my moment of truth had arrived. Time to step it up; time to share this experience and help others understand how to give themselves their best poker hand, or as Doctor George Bartzokis told me, "Better Odds"!

I have been there with you; I like to think of the boomer demographic as my people, our tribe. We are all in this together. My story of insecurities and the fallout of the so-called nuclear family we were all raised in, carries many similarities with other boomers. I am sure many will be able to relate.

This book is by a boomer – and I'm damn proud of it. Born in 1959, one of 4,295,000, the bulk of my boomer brothers and sisters are just a little bit older than me. Frankly, I always looked up to you older people. I always envied my friends who had older brothers and sisters; being the oldest of a tribe of five, I wished I had someone to plow the way in life ahead of me.

In school, the teachers always remembered your family name, your older siblings, and your parents. I, on the other hand, was a lone wolf, who had to cut the cake on my own. I was very shy and insecure as a young child. Insecurities did not ever help in the '60s; this personality trait had to go away if you ever wanted to make any friends. I always thought the older kids were so very cool. I was jealous and timid. Insecure? Oh, yes. My insecurity has fueled my life and personality, and has actually made me a stronger person (it took therapy to figure that out), but hey, nothing's wrong with that.

So why read another self-help book? There are hundreds, if not thousands in print, so what makes this one so much better, or even different?

You are going to find this a very different read: a life story by a boomer, for boomers; a way to move forward in what I like to call the "Indian summer" of our lives. Examples of goals achieved, finishing unfinished business (yes, I was a college dropout; more insecurity), illustrations and motivation (always battling weight issues, insecurities), that worked for me and that I know can work for you. Being ordinary has its advantages; I should know.

I am there with all of you, my brother and sister boomers who are looking around this world we live in and wondering, "How in the hell did life run off the rails? And now what?" We did it right, we paid our dues, we invented things, built a dynasty, laid the foundation for our children, and now...?

We watched a man walk on the moon, we listened to the Beatles, and we experienced Disco. Elvis was the "King" and rock and roll exploded. We invented walking on the edge.

My dad loved the Honeymooners and Sinatra; I loved The Doobies and The Flintstones. He watched Gunsmoke and sang Perry Como; we had the Beverly Hillbillies and Pink Floyd. He listened to Herb Alpert and the Tijuana Brass; we had KC and the Sunshine Band. He drove an Oldsmobile; I wanted a Firebird or a Camaro.

We find that the programmed future, the end of the rainbow, the "Golden Years" are not our parents' world; we want more, much more, because things turned out a lot different. We learn that the future is fluid, that in order to maintain what you will read all through this book, what I refer to as QOL (quality of life), change and adaptation are inevitable.

Believe me, I get the pain, I've been through the turmoil, and I watched my parents divorce when I was in high school in the seventies. I then lived through my own divorce in the eighties, had a drinking issue, abused drugs, and struggled with self-identity. I had the near death experience, went back to college as an older adult, and struggled as a single parent.

My life did not end; it is just beginning. Yours can, too!

I have so many issues, yet they all fuel my passion. The world is evolving, and changing, and so much for the better—you just have to believe.

This book is a blessing; it is a map and a recipe to share with all of you who feel alone and isolated, who think that the best days are behind you, when in fact you hold the keys to the best days that are yet to come. We all just need a reboot of our mentality, a chance to remember who we are: the pioneers, the hippies of the sixties, the rockers of the seventies, and the entrepreneurs and leaders throughout the twentieth century. We made America great, and it is time to step up and with our collective voice, live the lives that we deserve and have earned.

But you have to have a map, and this book is just that: a map to show you how an ordinary boomer decided to take a stand and change his life, and then go out and show everyone how he did it.

It is all true, and it really did work, and is working still, and together we ROCK, as in "Boomers Rock"!

My overriding wish is to do work that is significant and beneficial to others. The hand of God is guiding me, metaphorically speaking, like Adam Smith's "Invisible Hand". He guides everything that is occurring in my life: the business, the radio show, the website, my education, and of course the dream, to help others through examples and guiding principles that will work to change our mindsets.

It is critical to articulate why this matters. The goal is creating and fueling passion in numbers, to reach a tipping point, which will then create real change in the world. Fitness, nutrition, and positive thinking—the foundational principles of an improved quality of life— have been treated as fads in America for the past 100 years. When people figure out how best to improve all three of those principles at the same time, the improved quality of life will sustain those principles in their daily life. When enough people improve their quality of life, the habits become ingrained and fads become a move- ment. And a movement that improves lives becomes

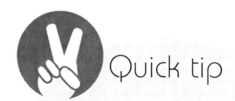

Quick tip

Hit the gym instead of happy hour. Drinking alcohol immediately after feeling stress (like, for example, 30 minutes after work) can block the hormone cortisol, which results in an increase in stress. A workout is a guaranteed stress beater. And a workout doesn't have to be any- thing huge—any movement (espe- cially walking) is great!

self-sustaining. The Baby Boomers are poised to turn fads into a movement. They are "Boomers who Rock"!

People today are ravenous for positive recognition and positive reinforcement, but most of us, for whatever reason, are not receiving it. The time has come to change that mindset and perception. An old friend and professor once told me: "Always re-create yourself, be willing to look forward to change and learn something new every day." At that point I didn't get it, didn't understand; it took growing up and going back to school—in my forties—to understand the principle. You have the chance to change your demeanor every day; that's the beauty of life. However, our minds are clouded by issues and perceptions of gloom.

Waking up every day and doing an affirmation of some sort will kick start your mindset. Invent new ways to build enthusiasm for life, and never rest on your laurels. When you live in the greatest country in the world, during the best times in history, understand me when I tell you that through adversity grows opportunity. It amazes me that many people fail to realize what we have. If we all had a chance to see how the majority of the world lives, we would seize every opportunity we have here in the U.S.

> He who has health, has hope; he who has hope, has everything.
>
> ~Old Arabian Proverb

2: Ponce de Leon

Ponce de Leon and his story of the search for the fountain of youth provided an interesting topic to begin this book, and I wanted to share a touch of his story before throwing the 21st century spin on it. First Ponce...

The story of the "Fountain of Youth" has been around for millennia. Tales of such a fountain have been told across the world for thousands of years. It was Ponce de Leon that many of us remember from school as the 16th century explorer of what is now Florida.

I find it ironic now to see Florida as the bastion of snow-birds and retirees seeking refuge from the cruel northern winter as the site where Ponce hoped to make his discovery. History has it several ways, but it is reported that nowhere in de Leon's writings did he mention the actual "quest" for the fountain of youth.

Again, in the ironies of ironies, Ponce had his conquests and successes, and like so often today the ephemeral feeling of success can be fleeting. Sailing with Columbus in his second voyage in 1493, Ponce was on the fast track to stardom. Settling with his family on what is now known as the Dominican Republic, he became a military commander and deputy governor.

In 1506, Ponce discovered a nearby island named Borinquen, now called Puerto Rico. Through great fortune, success would again smile on Ponce as he discovered large deposits of gold. Realizing he had the break of his lifetime he left to share his good fortune. He returned to Borinquen in 1508 on orders of the King of Spain to colonize and explore the new land, and was named governor of the island. De Leon had the good life—for a short time, that is. As it turns out, and as happens for so many people in life's cruel turn of events (promotions passing you by, political wheeling and dealings), Ponce was replaced as governor two years later by none other than Columbus's son.

After plummeting from the high of conquest, discovery, and becoming a Spanish rock star, de Leon set sail, hurt by the King's action, in search of new treasure. He had heard of a legendary "fountain of youth." Indians spoke of a magical spring whose water was believed to make older people young again. Ponce de León explored many areas, including the Bahamas and Bimini, for both gold and the mythical fountain, and in March of 1513 his ships landed on Florida's east coast near present-day St. Augustine. He claimed the land he named La Florida (LAH flow REE dah), the "place of flowers", for the King of Spain.

De Leon would continue his quest and search for fortune and the mythical fountain of youth for many years, exploring many areas of Florida until he decided to build a permanent camp in 1521 on the white sandy beaches of the Gulf of Mexico. It was here that he was eventually ambushed by Indians, sustaining a serious arrow wound to his leg. Deciding that this may not be the most ideal place to build a settlement the group, led by de Leon, fled back to Cuba where he succumbed to his injury and died; he was 61.

He will always be remembered as the brave conquistador who first explored many parts of Florida, but as history has been written de Leon may have been in search for more than fortune. His zest for the fountain of youth may have come from an ulterior motive. It is reported that Ponce de León was looking for the waters of Bimini to cure his impotence.

The quest for the "Fountain of Youth" and riches that led to Ponce de Leon's eventual death is so similar to the love affair that American society has with this image of looking back, fantasizing about our youth. This constant focus on issues that are unreachable, and irrelevant, has led to a functional demise of sorts. It has established this mindset of the days of youth being the best of life, and quite frankly, this is wrong. Looking back to reminisce is one thing; trying to be something we are not is completely another. That is where I am coming from with this book.

Boomers, our best days are ahead of us. The story you are going to read in this book will show you how to accomplish the goals that will enable a magnificent future, describe the necessary tools to enhance and energize, the education and knowledge only gleaned from living life to the fullest and understanding how to maintain, improve and regain energy levels that you may think have long since left you.

Pull meaning from your life, use that knowledge NOT to regain the so called "fountain", but to improve the future and use the wisdom acquired through the years to achieve a special existence full of meaning, health, and happiness. Make every day special and remember it is one step forward to a better life.

"The 200% Solution" is a winning formula because we can work effectively, congenially, and productively with all ages. We as boomers need to embrace this, and learn from the younger generations, so that we can establish a system of learning from each other, developing a synergy of teamwork. That's what our mission is all about: everyone becoming successful, because we are all talented in some way.

3: The '60s—
What a decade!

Growing up as a child in the '60s was sometimes difficult. My parents, I believe, were similar to many other young people that decade. They had married young, in the late fifties, with all of the fifties styles and mentalities: "I Love Lucy", or "The Honeymooners", or "Father Knows Best". I bet many of my boomer brothers' and sisters' parents were the same, had the same problems and wound up in the same boat: young, not ready for parenthood and looking for an escape from the tyranny of their own parents. The only way out was getting married, so it was normal. My mother was very young, only 16 years old. At 17 she had me; at 18, my brother; and at 20, my sister—three children and she wasn't even 21. Poor young woman, she did not have a clue as to the hellions she

had coming; in the '60s it was a different era. My dad
was only five years older than she, so he had his hands
full just trying to make a living and feed his kids.

We moved around a lot when I was very young—I
mean a lot, almost like a military family. It did not bode
well for my parents' relationship; it laid the foundation
for a rocky situation. Dad was a draftsman, working on
naval ship drawings, so we lived in some faraway locations; we moved several times by the time I started
school. I think that was where my insecurities started,
being the oldest, and not really putting down roots. It
was hard on us, but dad did what he thought was best,
and was pretty good at his job, so new offers were always coming in. And the ability to move around the
country was a relatively new phenomenon; remember
the highway system was built right around this time
in history, and people were becoming mobile, cars were
plentiful, and gas was 31 cents a gallon.

By the time I started school in 1965 we had moved
three times. We went from the west coast (San Diego),
to the Deep South (New Orleans, Louisiana, and Pas-
cagoula, Mississippi) for naval work. My sister was
actually born in New Orleans in 1962, during—of all
things—Mardi Gras. We finally landed in Bay City,
Michigan, where I would spend most of my elementary years and gain two new brothers. Before my mom
was 27 years old she had five children, standard stuff
for those turbulent times. Five kids, young parents,
one income. I give my folks credit; it had to have been
rough—no wonder their marriage was always borderline dysfunctional, which frankly did not help my
personal insecurities. But hey, they did for us, provided as best they could, and we were a great bunch for
the most part; my parents loved their children, even
though they didn't like each other very much.

The 1960s were a turbulent time; looking back I think it started the conditioning for what we now call the information society, and the fast-paced lives we live today. People think that we have it rough today; well, let's talk about some of the issues of the '60s.

The decade of the Vietnam War began with what is probably not thought of much today, but in retrospect was huge: the first televised presidential debates. Today we are bombarded with media, appearances of politicians, social media and radio talk shows. However, it was the 1960s that brought Kennedy and Nixon, and television probably won the election for JFK. Even though Nixon was an older, more experienced politician, with the brain power to back up his positions, he did not look good on black and white TV—remember that sweaty upper lip? With JFK's coolness and boyish handsomeness, he had the look of a movie star and those debates got him elected.

Did you catch the black and white TV line?

Yes, black and white TV, and then color television came to our house in the late '60s and believe me it was a HUGE DEAL! We were one of the first on our block, and even though there was not much programming in color, it didn't matter; it was color. Sunday nights with Disney and "Bonanza" were awesome.

Black and white television ruled, heck—having any kind of programming was great, even though you never watched TV during the day; we had what was called "get outside and play" as the mantra, those nights when you did watch television brought a new sense of fun and laughter to our lives. We had the premiers of such shows as the "Flintstones"; as the first primetime cartoon in 1960, Fred and Wilma broke new ground being the first animated program to actually show the opposite sex sleeping together—the audacity and outrage!

The "Flintstones" premiered on September 30, 1960, and ran for four years—166 episodes in all. Until the "Simpsons" came along, Fred, Barney, Wilma, Betty, Bam-Bam, Pebbles, and of course, Dino, were the kings of primetime animated television. The "Munsters", "The Addams Family", "Gilligan's Island" and the "Jetsons"... and, of course, my dad's favorite: "The Honeymooners" with Jackie Gleason, set the stage for future generations of sitcoms and cartoons. No list would be complete without the biggest show of them all: "The Beverly Hillbillies", which ran from 1962-65 in black and white and was then produced in color from 1965-71 because it was such a huge hit. BH was the number one show in America twice, and ran for nine seasons with a mind-blowing 274 episodes.

Drama was big in the '60s, with Alfred Hitchcock scaring the crap out of us. With "Psycho" in 1960, starring Janet Leigh, (yes Jamie Lee Curtis's mom), and Tipi Hendren in "The Birds", I was fascinated by Alfred, who had his own television show, too—he was big, really big. Star Trek premiered in 1966, and what young boy did not love the female crew with those short skirts? Come to think of it, I had several television crushes, between Mary Ann on "Gilligan", Barbara Eden on "I Dream of Jeanie" (1965), and Ellie Mae on "The Beverly Hillbillies", I couldn't make up my mind; they were all dolls. "Batman", "Bewitched", "Dragnet", "Gunsmoke", "Mission Impossible", "The Rat Patrol" , "Mr. Ed" (how would a show about a talking horse work today?), and last but not at all least, "The Andy Griffith Show" with little Ronnie Howard. I think we grew up with Ron; television brought us together for the good times, and unfortunately, the bad.

We lost our President in 1963 to an assassin's bullet, and it was replayed over and over on television. Great men were killed, like Martin Luther King, Jr. and Bobby Kennedy, and riots ensued in Los Angeles in 1965 and Detroit in 1968. We lived through the Six Day War, the Bay of Pigs, and the Cuban Missile Crisis, and meanwhile the Berlin Wall was erected and we "ducked and covered" as the Cold War became a part of us. We sent young American men to war in Vietnam in 1965; many perished, and the daily count on Walter Cronkite's CBS evening news was a daily reminder that young people were dying, and global turmoil and anxiety was constantly omnipresent, even for a little boy. Thank goodness we had sitcoms and the "Beatles", "GI Joe" and a new bicycle; the sixties conditioned us to become who we are today: the boomers of the 21st century. We adapt and grow; it's called life.

4: Moving forward

So what, in fact, is it that gives a person the desire for change? What possesses a woman to climb a mountain, fly in a spaceship or compete in a triathlon? What drives a man to run with bulls, recreate his professional life, or break the four-minute mile? What is it?

Those are the questions I kept asking myself, over and over, as my notes for this book continued to grow.

I believe I have found an answer. Throughout my own life, so many wonderful things continued to occur that I needed to synthesize the whole process, step back and break things down and get the "recipe" for success and reinvention.

What I found was this: it is a logical combination of many different things. Logical? Okay, so why, in all of the books, in all the articles, lectures and discussions, different ingredients of the recipe to success and achievement of dreams and goals are discussed but not fully explained? The answer is this: it's the combination; it's the ratio— the right mix in the right order—that has been missing all along. All of the components have been around for a long time; it is just that we never had exactly the right combination. It took Edison more than 1,000 attempts to finally get his light bulb to work. One thousand!

So okay, enough, what is this breakthrough that has eluded the scholars and experts?

It's The 200% Solution!

Jim Collins, in his bestseller, Good to Great , spoke about the enemy of great. The enemy of great is good. The problem is that we have good schools, not great, that we have good government, not great, and so on. So few bother to push the envelope to greatness that we have become soft and accept good, as good enough. And actually, as technology has improved our lives we have gone from good to average, and even in some cases become the consummate underachievers. Yikes!

I know I was leading the pack of couch potatoes, and finally the moment of truth woke this potato up (more on that later).

And that is where my 200% formula comes from.

I needed to push myself to achieve the goals and dreams that I wanted, to increase both my choice and my accountability. It was turning the dream into a habit, a goal into an accomplishment; that was the end result.

And that is where 200% was born.

As you read this book, understand that most, if not all, of the lessons, drills, beliefs and actions were my way of changing. Through the actions and behaviors, changes and tips I do or have done, still, to this day, on a daily basis, I am my own personal guinea pig. That's why I am so passionate about sharing the recipe, the lifestyle and the story. When you make the decision to end the couch potato disease it is a lifelong commitment, and oh so worth it, so I thank you for reading this far, and thank you for even thinking about improving your life; it really is the first ingredient in our lifestyle recipe that is 200%: DESIRE!

I was given a second chance by a higher power, and part of my agreement with the big man upstairs is sharing, and teaching.

Studies have shown that retirement has its risks, specifically to our brain health. Retirement often takes us out of the game of life: that engaging, stimulating, socially integrated part of living that can keep our brains functioning at an optimal level. We need to maintain what is known as our "cognitive capacity," our brain's well of backup systems that we all too often take for granted. Age-related brain issues (much more on that later) tend to make themselves apparent as we enter the "Golden Years."

Just as in the old saying in athletics, "Use it or lose it," our brains have been shown to be much more like a muscle than ever before. The sooner you understand the "how" to do this, the "why" will become very apparent.

I propose that it is not just maintaining what we have that is important (millions of boomers are demonstrating that fact clearly with their renewed zest for life), but that there are many ways to completely improve what I will refer to often as QOL (quality of life). It will be through staying in the forefront, finding what you love to do, learning new skills through intellectually stimulating activities, and staying socially integrated and busy that will build our life expectancies and therefore our QOL.

Just as you need a financial fitness plan, you need a mental game plan, and that is what this book will do—

provide you with the information and tips that have worked for others, helping them regain zest and great numbers physical fitness (I am talking referring to all of the blood work stuff, weight, and body-fat).

Improving your quality of life should not be a struggle; if you are not satisfied with your state of being, then throw your habits out the window.

This is not a self-improvement book that will tell you what to do, so much as show you how to do it. Since many of the examples are firsthand, I felt that compelling pull to share the experience. Even though I thought I had made a decision to just improve my own life after almost buying the farm... or kicking the bucket—the more I became a different person, through mindset, nutrition and fitness changes, the more it became clear what the purpose of my life was becoming.

I never had a clue as far as this messenger business goes, and it is the culmination of many events: recovering from illness, improving my health, finishing college, starting our business, placing in the body building show, developing the website and now delivering the radio talk show—the sense of purpose was overwhelming.

Writing this book is a leap of faith; however, bucket lists grow, and learning about improving brain skills, through many interviews and readings, definitely lit the fire.

Are you ready? Is your head in the right direction? The 200% Solution is broken down into three sections:

110% is your brain—the physiology and the behavior that define your being. Treating your brain well is the best thing you can do for yourself.

60% is food—what you put in your engine, the amounts, and the time of day all contribute to your success. Feed your brain, feed your body, and create a positive feedback loop between them that will propel you forward.

30% is activity—finding what you love to do, joining your tribe, and enjoying the social side of life and health. Whether it's sports fitness, social activities, or just playing games, the physical movement you love is the one you should do.

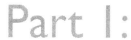

Part I:

YOUR BRAIN (110%)

Here is an athletic analogy to start off the brain section of the book. Think of it this way: If a running back has to hit the hole; if a gymnast must nail the flip; if the swimmer wins the race; the academic publishes the paper; what is the one thing that everyone has to do first? Let me tell you. It is getting your head moving in the right direction, because you will never accomplish your goal without this principle. Get your head right, thinking right, moving in the right positive direction and anything is possible, anything! Now let's talk about that wonderful machine inside our head: our brain.

As we boomers continue to understand that life, the way we decide to live, and the quality of that life is more and more in our control, one thing became exceedingly clear: We are not our parents, and we are going to live our lives in a completely different way than they did. This pre-programmed "age", 65, is no longer applicable to us, and we want more, much more. Life expectancy is expanding; the potential to live well into our 80s, 90s and the centenarian magic number of 100 is becoming more and more a reality.

If longevity continues to proliferate, which undoubtedly it will, having an understanding of how to maintain our brain health is paramount.

Being in the telecom industry for what seems like forever (almost 30 years as of this writing), having been through the middle of the greatest advancements in technological history with the advent of digital communications, which led to the proliferation of the Internet, I have been acutely aware of technological change. Couple that with my academic background, which gave me a very solid foundation of history, policy, growth and management, I am keenly aware of how our telecommunications growth in the United States has led to advancements never imagined; we have become a network-based world, and believe me—it's only going to continue to speed up in the 21st century.

I have grown to find brain health, the internal networks of our body's communication system, the central nervous system, to have very strong parallels with the history of the telephone and internet technologies.

When comparing Alexander Graham Bell's invention of the telephone in 1876 with the way the brain works, the networking functions of both are eerily similar.

I love using analogies and metaphors to paint pictures of how I see things, so as we move forward in understanding the importance of our brain and its functions, you will notice how I draw parallels to both. It should be fun and interesting at the same time.

Communication technologies have driven innovation and education, and made the world flat, as Thomas Freedman wrote in his book of the same title. Pictures on cave walls, the written word, printing presses, books, radio, telephone, television, computing, educational and technological innovations, can be compared to the philosophies of medical care, practical understanding, thought, behavior, learning, mental health, localizationist theory, brain plasticity... and the list continues to expand. That is the point as the world moves faster, and theories and practices never imagined become common; it really is amazing.

There are major issues with longer life, and the first key to maintaining that magic QOL is our brain health.

So living longer is entirely possible—more like probable—fantastic! We all need to get a grip on how and what we have inside our heads, and understand its functionality, and how to protect our beautiful minds. Moving forward into our "golden years" without the full capacity and understanding of how to exercise and keep our brains young and functioning will leave us all at risk of—at worst—dementia and Alzheimer's, or – at best—fixed in the thought processes and behaviors that made our parents old before their time; it is our choice.

This is where the importance of the 200% action plan comes into focus: that 110% of our well-being, our quality of life, is completely dependent upon how our brains function and maintain the physiological vitality, which then leads to our subconscious and conscious behaviors.

Think of it as understanding how our machinery works, the "what", which then leads to the "how".

The key is understanding the limitless potential for change. How we perceive, the intrinsic perception of our existence, is directly related to our brain and how the processes and functionality take place. We need to understand how our brain creates imagination, dreams, attitudes, behaviors, goals, faith; where it all happens and what makes change completely possible. Our acceptance and maintenance of our own health, working at the levels of growth and never giving up on growing are the keys to our brain health, which in turn is the key to our physical health and our existence. It is the "you can do it" mentality that boomers now must grasp and embrace. Our brains are dynamic and exceedingly powerful, the most prolific and awesome power ever imagined, and they are continually ready to grow, change and absorb material and learn all of the sensory inputs that we experience. Your brain is an unbelievable and limitless powerhouse machine!

With over 100 billion neurons we possess unlimited potential, a "universe inside our brains", with 100,000 miles of blood vessels, and where 25% of our blood flow is used, 20% of our oxygen consumed, 30% of the water we drink and over 40% of all nutrients we consume; our brains rule supreme in our body.

Everything starts and ends with our brain.

We owe all of the understanding of this knowledge of our brains' unlimited power to doctors over the last 500 years. Their lives were committed to understanding how we learn, process information, and the coordination of reflex and non-reflex action, dreams, behaviors and illness.

I admire healthcare professionals, researchers, and doctors more than you can imagine. The amount of time and effort they invest in their professions is incredible. Healthcare work is demanding and difficult, and it takes special people to work in that industry. I have made the comment around the house many times about healthcare being "Production Work"; harsh, but in my opinion true.

The changes that we as boomers are going to see in our "healthcare" (I could go off on a tangent here and bring up Paul Zane Pilzner's Wellness Revolution—more on that another time), are likely to bring us closer and closer to that "production healthcare." This type of assembly line service is going to be a major driver in the years to come, and will especially affect us boomers.

It is up to us to get our heads moving in that direction, the self-accountability and self-maintenance of our own well-being that will deliver that QOL. Understanding my 200% plan and its components is the key to success, and it all begins with our brains. The research, interviews, studying of our physical and mental conditions which govern the "neuro" field is amazingly enlightening. The people who have dedicated their lives to this field of study are incredible.

I especially want to express my admiration for the Neurologists, Psychiatrists, Neuroscientists, Psychologists, and research assistants, as this field of study and practice is tough. The work is tedious, and many times the patients and their issues, illnesses and cases are very severe and take years to work through. It takes a special quality of person to continue to work through this, and we as the human race owe these wonderful people a debt of gratitude, because without the years of work and research they have done, many people would not be living better, more meaningful lives. For that, I want to thank them.

In this section of the book we will discuss two prima-ry schools of thought: the physical side of brain health and processes, which includes the physiological compo-nents that make up our neurology and nervous system; and the behavioral aspects that are derived from the physical. I found it so exciting to research and talk to healthcare specialists, authors and experts about this topic, and it became exceedingly clear that the 110% of the 200% plan devoted to our mind and behaviors is by far the most important aspect of improving our quality of life (QOL).

Both the physiological and behavioral aspects are im-portant, and a solid education about the "how and why", along with the "who, what, where and when", is the key to the beginning of everything that can be brought about in our quest to improve. That QOL has several key in-gredients is a given; however, it is in the order laid out in the 200% plan that will truly work if you follow and adapt these beliefs and mindsets.

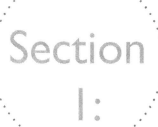

Section I:

Brain Physiology

> The ultimate measure of a man is not where he stands in moments of comfort but where he stands at times of challenge and controversy.
>
> ~Rev. Dr. Martin Luther King, Jr.

Our bodies are made up of networks, which adapt and grow, always changing and trying to improve. The unlimited potential for improvement is so exciting; and it is, and has been, and will continue to be, so much fun to encounter. Sometimes when I talk to these special people on the radio show, or read their books, I truly feel like a kid in a candy store. It is my ambition to share this "map" with everyone so that you can enjoy the benefits the "candy", because frankly, sharing is what it is all about.

> Courage is not the absence of fear, but rather the judgment that something else is more important than fear.
>
> ~Ambrose Redmoon

5: Courage Means Overcoming Fear

Like ingredients of a great recipe, each of my suggestions to you has its own redeeming quality, and each should be taken on its own merit. They have been drawn from many different sources. In essence the recipe, or road map, can be different for each person, a unique process of getting from point A to point B, or making your own flavor; it's up to you to decide.

In reality, we all have our lives, and the accountability for achievement of our dreams and goals falls strictly on our own shoulders. In a way, to use a computer analogy, there are countless different ways to get to the same result, so use whatever you find comfortable for you. That is why I have many suggestions; there is no one-size-fits all here—you are who you are, and this book is what it is: suggestions to people I care about—just like the radio show—suggestions, affirmations, ideas and examples.

Who says you cannot re-invent yourself? Can a person recreate, or reincarnate their life? Is there an age at which this is no longer possible? Think about it this way:

Trainer T's rule of human adaptability: Where the refrigerator door (your RAS) meets passion, there develops the physical and physiological change, brain change (neurogenesis, neuroplasticity and myelin), to make the process of adaptation work. Don't worry—this sounds deep and complicated at first, but it's really exciting.

The "Law of Attraction" does put you in the right place mentally. It is through a hybrid model (I have always loved hybrids; in the telecom industry hybrids were key first-movers in the shift to the information age, um... digress, um... well, yeah), where positive energy is just a component of fulfillment in conjunction with the "Law".

However, this process will not occur on its own. You not only need focus (remember, "laser-like" focus), and effort (and lots of it), but an additional catalyst is needed for the reaction to start. It begins as a mental phenomenon but must move into a physical arena; the continuation is an individual formula, because everyone is unique; however, I believe the steps are always very similar. It is your own version of your "recipe" for fulfillment in your life that will hold the key to success.

I now know that something has guided me to this point in my life, something that has been pushing my sail, for so long unbeknownst to me, to become what I am now: the messenger. I was a single dad in my early thirties, making bad decisions (like a lot of young adults). Then giving up drinking in my thirties, going back to college at forty, getting married at 41 (for the second time), doing a body building show at 50, becoming a talk show host at 51... who would have thunk it? Even during the darkest days of daily alcohol abuse, recreational drug use, and a rudderless journey, something helped me to reconnect with the girl of my dreams 25 years after dating in high school. It really has always been God's plan to send me on this grandest of journeys.

That, I am now completely sure of!

I am also sure of these truths: That the journey into the tunnel of darkness does have a redeeming quality after all: hope! That anyone who enters the tunnel, or who is now in the tunnel, or someone who is just wandering in a tunnel of despair should fear not; there does exist the light at the end, and it will be your life events that will ultimately lead you to that light. It is the hope and energy of positive thinking and never quitting that will guide you. It has made me appreciate my journey and my mindset is now clear; to appreciate and emulate, to invigorate and educate many with a willingness to share the plight. It is a daily journey to find oneself. Though the information in this book is solid, fundamental, and logical, it is not rocket science and it is really nothing new, just a different perspective, through a different lens, from a different voice. Anyone and everyone can benefit from some or all of my story, the message and the tips you will derive from this book.

I do try and "narrow cast" on the radio show; with the current format of one hour it's done really quickly, so in that forum it is "Get the message out," for the most part to "Boomers" and listeners to the program. And let me make it abundantly clear how blessed I feel to have the honor to share the message over the FTNS network. Whatever happens in the future, I will always remember where the radio show started. Like a phoenix, the vision of multimedia and sharing the core values and beliefs of health and wellness has always been in my dream.

6: The Physiology: Brain Health Is Everything!

While the great, deep-thinking distinction between mind and body in Western thought can be traced to the Greeks, it is to the groundbreaking work of René Descartes (1596-1650), French mathematician, philosopher, and physiologist, that we owe the first logical account of the mind/body relationship.

Descartes was born in Touraine in the small town of La Haye, and was educated from the age of eight at the Jesuit college of La Flèche. And we owe the diffusion of this knowledge to Guttenberg.

A philosopher and a goldsmith; strange bedfellows, that is for certain.

At La Flèche, Descartes formed the habit of spending the morning in bed, engaged in systematic meditation. During his meditations, he was struck by the sharp contrast between the certainty of mathematics and the controversial nature of philosophy, and came to believe that the sciences could be made to yield results as certain as those of mathematics.

In this work, Descartes proposed a mechanism for automatic reaction in response to external events. According to his proposal, external motions affect the peripheral ends of the nerve fibrils, which in turn displace the central ends. As the central ends are displaced, the pattern of interfibrillar space is rearranged and the flow of animal spirits is thereby directed into the appropriate nerves.

It was Descartes' articulation of this mechanism for automatic, differentiated reaction that led to his generally being credited with the founding of reflex theory. By focusing on the problem of true and certain knowledge, Descartes had made epistemology, the question of the relationship between mind and world, the starting point of philosophy.

By localizing the soul's contact with the body in the pineal gland, Descartes had raised the question of the relationship of mind to the brain and nervous system. Yet at the same time, by drawing a radical ontological (Greek, for the nature of being), distinction between body as extended and mind as pure thought, Descartes, in search of certitude, had paradoxically created intellectual chaos.

Interesting, the relationship (or timing in history might be a better term) of Descartes' philosophical beliefs and the invention of the printing press. If education and the diffusion of ideas are keys to getting your head right, then I would be remiss not to mention the printed word and its diffusion of information.

Networks, education, and knowledge, oh my! These do a brain good.

The printing press was invented by Guttenberg around 1440. A goldsmith by profession, he developed a complete printing system, which perfected the printing process through all its stages by adapting existing technologies to printing purposes, as well as making groundbreaking inventions of his own. He devised a tool, the "hand mold", which for the first time made possible the precise and rapid creation of metal movable type in large quantities, a key element in the profitability of the whole printing enterprise.

The mechanization of bookmaking led to the first mass production of books in history in assembly style. A single Renaissance period printing press could produce 3,600 pages per workday, compared to forty by typographic hand style. Books of bestselling authors like Luther or Erasmus were sold by the hundreds of thousands in their lifetime.

From a single point of origin, Mainz, Germany, printing spread within several decades to over two hundred cities in a dozen European countries. By 1500, printing presses in operation throughout Western Europe had already produced more than twenty million volumes.

In the 16th century, with presses spreading further afield, their output rose tenfold to an estimated 150 to 200 million copies. The operation of a press became so synonymous with the enterprise of printing that it lent its name to an entire new branch of media.

As early as 1620, the English statesman and philosopher Sir Francis Bacon could write that typographical printing has "changed the whole face and state of things throughout the world".

7: The Nervous System: An Overview

Our nervous system is our internal network; it is where everything begins and ends. It is the mode of transport of the electrical impulses from receptor sites to our brain, and the transferring of the information, processing of those signals, and the return trip back to our muscles and skeletal system. It is the beginning of our everyday living. It is important to put the pieces together to form the basis for our improvement, reaching our QOL; after all, journeys are always easier if you have a map, and you understand the route.

The nervous system is a collection of billions of cells forming the nerves that

are specifically designed to provide our internal communication network. It is the central command center
that collects and gathers information about our internal
and external environments.

The three primary functions of our nervous system
are the sensory, motor, and integrative. The sensory
function is our ability to sense change in the internal
environment (stretching a muscle for example), and the
external environment, (walking on a slippery surface).
The motor function is our reaction (muscular or nervous
systems response) to sensory input, for example adjust-
ing our walking pattern when the surface is slippery.
And the integrative function is the ability to interpret
the stimulus and make decisions and respond.

The key is to understand that all movement, thoughts,
decisions, and learning is directly dictated by our nervous system's ability to communicate with the control
center (our brain), and that without this electrical input
our brain cannot make a correct response, decision, or
adjustment. In a sense, the information superhighway
(the nervous system), without excellent routes, smooth
roads, and great rest areas, can make for a precarious
sensory informational journey to the brain.

Our nervous system is comprised of two interdepen-
dent divisions; think of cooperation to the highest degree between two similar entities. These divisions are
the peripheral nervous system, the side roads, neighborhood streets and backwoods trails to get us to the
end destination; and the central nervous system, the
major highway of our bodies, which is connected to command central, (our brain).

From a top view, notice how the brain is divided into
two halves, called hemispheres. Each hemisphere com-
municates with the other through the corpus callosum,

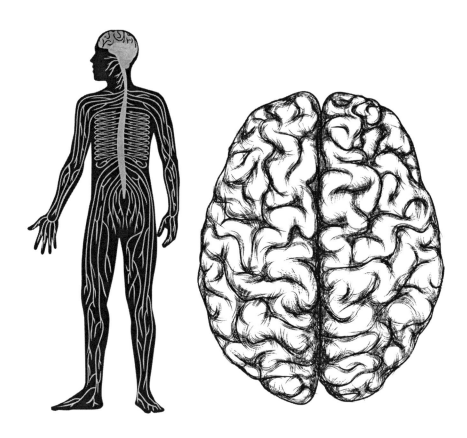

a bundle of nerve fibers. (Another smaller fiber bundle that connects the two hemispheres is called the anterior commissure).

Some differences between the peripheral nervous system (PNS) and the central nervous system (CNS):

1. In the Central Nervous System, collections of neurons are called nuclei. In the Peripheral Nervous System, collections of neurons are called ganglia.

2. In the Central Nervous System, collections of axons are called tracts. In the PNS, collections of axons are called nerves.

In the peripheral nervous system, neurons can be functionally divided in three ways:

1. Sensory (afferent)—carry information TOWARD the central nervous system from sense organs or motor (efferent)—carry information AWAY FROM the central nervous system (for muscle control).

2. Cranial—connects the brain with the periphery, or Spinal—connects the spinal cord with the periphery.

3. Somatic—connects the skin or muscle with the central nervous system, or Visceral—connects the internal organs with the central nervous system.

For many years the study of brain science was very limited, still following Descartes' philosophies, and it was not until Dr. Wilder Penfield of the Montreal Neurological Institute in the 1930s began his research into "mapping", which started to unravel the nervous system's integration into our command center.

Wilder Penfield (1891 – 1976): "The Organ of Destiny"

Wilder Penfield was born in Spokane, Washington, and spent much of his youth in Hudson, Wisconsin. When he was 13, in 1904, his mother learned of the newly established Rhodes scholarship. "This is just the thing for you," he recalled his mother saying with great confidence. To win, he would have to become an all-round scholar athlete. "The fact that my mind was really that of a plodder, and that my gangling body was slow and awkward, would be, it seemed, no obstacle whatever." But he accepted the challenge of this ambition, and preparing himself shaped the years to come. He went to Princeton University, not least because it was in the small state of New Jersey, and Rhodes Scholarships were awarded on a state-by-state basis. While there he decided to pursue medicine—the profession of his grandfather and estranged father—because it seemed the most direct way to "make the world a better place in which to live."

He did win the Rhodes scholarship after all, and spent years training at Oxford, and in Spain, Germany, and New York, before becoming the first neurosurgeon in Montreal. His driving goal was to establish a neurological institute, where surgeons, laboratory researchers, physiologists and all scientists in the field of neurology could work and share their knowledge. After a decade of fund raising and grant writing, he established the Montreal Neurological Institute in 1934.

In the 1950s, Penfield was trying to treat patients with intractable epilepsy. Before an epileptic seizure, he knew, patients experience an "aura", a warning that the seizure is about to occur. Penfield thought if he could provoke this aura with a mild electric current on the brain, then he would have located the source of the seizure activity and could remove or destroy that bit of tissue. While patients were fully conscious, though anesthetized, he opened their skulls and tried to pinpoint the source of their epilepsy.

His technique was often successful, but his experimental surgery led him to an even more dramatic discovery. Stimulation anywhere on the cerebral cortex could bring responses of one kind or another, but he found that only by stimulating the temporal lobes (the lower parts of the brain on each side) could he elicit meaningful, integrated responses such as memory, including sound, movement, and color. These memories were much more distinct than usual memory, and were often about things un-remembered under ordinary circumstances. Yet if Pen-field stimulated the same area again, the exact same memory popped up—a certain song, the view from a childhood window—each time. It seemed he had found a physical basis for memory, an "engram".

He also developed a map of the brain, often portrayed as a cartoon called the motor homunculus (miniature human being). This cartoon character has features drawn according to how much brain space they take up. Therefore, lips and fingers with their high number of nerve endings are larger than arms and legs.

Penfield was not only a groundbreaking researcher and devoted surgeon. During his life he was called "the greatest living Canadian". He devoted much thinking to the mystery of the mind, and continued until his death in 1976 to contemplate and question whether there is a scientific basis for the existence of the human soul[iii].

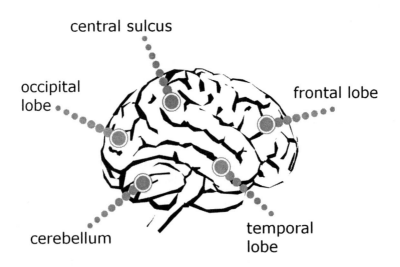

Until this study by Doctor Penfield, the actual operating system of our brain was still in its earliest understanding, and was referred to by the name "localizationist theory".

"Mapping" a person's brain in order to discover which parts of the body were represented in our brains, and how sensory inputs determined where the activities were processed, were the keys to the localizationist course of study, giving us our first glimpse or picture.

The localizationists had revealed that in our brain mapping the frontal lobes were the location of our motor system, which is responsible for initiating coordination of sensory inputs for the movement of our muscles. The three lobes behind the frontal lobe: the temporal, parietal, and occipital lobes, were the primary receptors and comprise our sensory system, which includes electrical signals sent from our sense sites: touch, ears, eyes, etc.

Of Dr. Penfield's greatest discoveries, one of the most significant was that our sensory and motor brain maps were similar to geographical maps, which emphasized adjacencies. Areas on the human body were generally next to each other on the brain maps. The really amazing fact is that when Dr. Penfield touched certain parts of the brain he discovered that he could trigger long-lost memories or dreamlike scenes in the test case, which led to the conclusion that higher mental activities were also mapped in the brain. Experts at the time assumed that the brain was unable to change and that these map locations and physical and behavioral tendencies were fixed.

Bell and the growth of another type of network

Alexander Graham Bell was born on March 3, 1847, in Edinburgh. He grew up deeply involved in the study of speech. He was also a talented musician able to play by ear from a very early age, and had he not been more interested in what his father was doing to help people speak, he might have ended up as a professional musician. He and his two brothers, an inventive trio, once built a model human skull and filled it with a good enough reproduction of the human vocal apparatus, which was worked with a bellows, so that it was reputed to be able to say, "Ma-ma."

Bell was twenty-nine years old when he received the patent on the telephone on March 7th, 1876, and it was also that same year that Edison invented the electric motor and phonograph. In 1877 Bell Telephone was started, which in 1878 had its first telephone listing with twenty-one people listed.

To use our brain and neural circuit/central nervous system analogy, the fetus was growing!

In three short years this new invention, the telephone, had morphed from an idea to over 30,000 circuits in use and the network of cables that we all take for granted. Telephone service being such an omnipresent utility, its birth and growth can be seen like our central nervous system and brain's development.

By 1890 the Bell System would have over 200,000 circuits in use, and as communication networks and inventions continued to proliferate in these amazing times, they, along with Guglielmo Marconi's invention of the radio, would become the foundation for the twentieth century's amazing growth. If you look at parallels, the end of the 19th century and the 20th century brought many astounding advancements that changed the way humans live their lives.

Here are some interesting human facts from the beginning of the 20th century.

In the year 1905:

- The average life expectancy in the U.S. was 47

- Only 14 percent of the homes in the U.S. had a bathtub

- There were only 8,000 cars in the U.S. and only 144 paved roads, and the maximum speed limit in most cities was 10 mph.

- More than 95 percent of all births in the U.S. took place at home

- Ninety percent of all U.S. physicians had no college education. Instead, they attended medical schools, many of which were condemned in the press, and were labeled by the government as "substandard."

- At a time when the average wage in the U.S. was 22 cents an hour, sugar cost four cents a pound. The average annual intake of refined sugar was 60 pounds per head, up from 7 pounds per head in 1805. (It was estimated to be about 150 pounds per head in 2005, a twenty-fold increase in just 200 years.)

- There were 230 reported murders in the entire U.S.

- Only 8 percent of homes had a telephone, and there were no computers, airplanes or 24-hour lighting.

Neurogenesis, plasticity, myelin; bits, bytes and networks

For 50 years our understanding of the brain was dominated by its rigid localization pattern. The common thought was that after a person's childhood the brain only changed when it began a long process of decline, when it failed to develop properly, or when it suffered an injury. It was believed that the brain could not alter its structure or functionality; that it was in fact "fixed or rigid." That is until another group of scientists began using tools and technologies that were actually developed in the 1930s, but not implemented until the late '70s; one of these tools is called MRI.

Magnetic resonance imaging, or scanning (also called an MRI), is a method of looking inside the body without using surgery, harmful dyes or x-rays. The MRI scanner uses magnetism and radio waves to produce clear pictures of the human anatomy. MRI is based on a physics phenomenon discovered in the 1930s, called nuclear magnetic resonance or NMR, in which magnetic fields and radio waves cause atoms to give off tiny radio signals. Felix Bloch, working at Stanford University, and Edward Purcell, from Harvard University, discovered NMR. NMR spectroscopy was then used as means to study the composition of chemical compounds.

This was followed by newer and more accurate brain scanning tools and technologies, which included single photon emission tomography (SPECT), positron emission tomography (PET), and magneto encephalography (MEG). The PET/CT scanner, attributed to physicist Dr. David Townsend and electrical engineer Dr. Ronald

Nutt, was named by TIME Magazine as the medical invention of the year in 2000.

With better diagnostic tools scientists and researchers were able to map the brain's electrical activity, and the clarity in which doctors could now visualize and rationalize concepts completely changed the world of neuroscience. Neuroscientists have estimated that over 90 percent of what we now know about the brain we have uncovered in the last fifteen to twenty years. The hardwired, fixed, rigid model, the "machine" that was thought to be the backbone of neuroscience, was now giving way to a new group of properties called neurogenesis, neuroplasticity, and of course myelin.

Learning how to learn

Neurogenesis, neuroplasticity, brain mapping, myelin, synapse growth, and mix a little bit of confidence plus the ever-present "passionate practice"; yes, those are some of the components you need to go back to college after more than twenty years. Let's not forget goals and dreams, plus the guts to walk into a classroom with over four hundred 18- to 21-year-olds... that was just the start of a long nine years, nine years that I would not change for anything.

Not that getting back into college in the first place was some cakewalk; they have what are called "standards" and "entrance requirements", which at first glance I did not meet.

I knew that the tanking at the end of my first stint in college in the early eighties was pretty awful, and once you get all of the transcripts from the four colleges I attended and then looked over the grades... sheesh, pretty good until that last semester, and then, well, let's say I was not Dean's List material; more like Animal House.

Dr. Wayne Dyer had some great comments on learning; he said there were two ways to become educated; they are:

1. Fear and doubt, which leads to the hard way of learning, suffering through your lessons, or

2. Absolute knowing, understanding that there is guidance available and you just have to reach out.

At first it was more the terror and then fear, which was closely followed by a ton of doubt; after that it was time to put my head down and just get going, and stop worrying about 'woulda, coulda, shoulda' stuff.

So it took sucking it up and asking for guidance, and it really is okay to ask for help. Once I got advice, went and did the "face-to-face" meeting with an admissions counselor (who obviously realized I was "non-traditional", which by the way is academic speak for "old guy"), and I explained the mission, and with my lifelong experience of being a dad, husband, etc., I was in. That's the thing: if you want something bad enough sometimes you have to go the extra mile. Did I say sometimes? Scratch that; you ALWAYS have to go the extra mile. No one gives anything of value for free; it just does not happen.

Setting goals is one thing, and it's great to get a pat on the back for a great idea, but now the real work begins: going to class, passing; time to re-learn how to learn.

TC 100: The first class

Marc Freedman's book "The Big Shift" is an extraordinary piece written for boomers by a boomer, a boomer I might add who has young children and has a great take on life. In his book he quotes Mary Catherine Bateson, anthropologist and writer, with this line that I just love:

"The doorway to this new stage of life is not filing for Social Security but thinking differently and continuing to learn."

I like it.

As boomers we have entered into this new phase, which is described many different ways, by many different names, including as University of Minnesota Sociologist Phyllis Moen, author of The Career Mystique called it, "midcourse", and as gerontologist Ken Dychtwald tags it, "middlescence".

Whatever flavor you want to color it, it is really up to you in essence. For me at this point it was called TERROR!

TC 100 is an entry level class in the telecommunication degree program at Michigan State University, which in essence means it is a cattle call. Four hundred plus students jam into an auditorium and get ready to learn. I was the student who was insecure and filled with anxiety, who lacked self-worth and self-confidence; plus the fact that I was the ugly duckling, middlescence, midcourse, midlife, old guy to traditional students... I think you catch my drift.

Oh, did I add clueless? As far as taking a class again, it was time to re-build my learning skills.

This is where the beauty of our beautiful brain comes into play, because our brains are always eager to take on new knowledge and skills, I had not learned of the phenomena of neurogenesis, plasticity and the function of myelin; I was going to memorize the textbook and write down every word my Professor said in lecture. Boy, I had a lot of myelin to build, but hey—the great thing is everyone has the time; it is just how to maximize the effort.

I now call it "Passionate Practice", however then it was just plain FEAR!

8: The '70s— Growing Up

The 1970s was a time of great growth, experience, learning and heartache. Looking back, if you think the second decade of the 21st century is a time of tremendous change, I don't think it holds a candle to the changes of the '70s; it was a very special time in the world.

As a family we finally stopped our nomadic moving. We changed schools once more and settled in Lansing, Michigan. In my six years of elementary school life I had attended five different schools, for the most part private Catholic schools, but due to family issues (remember my parents' disdain for each other) we for whatever reason continued to shift around. By now there were five children in our family; in 1970 we were 11, 10, 8, 5 and 2 years old. Of course I was the oldest, and still longing to have that older brother or sister to blaze the trail. Insecurities? Yes, there were plenty. I have to say that even though we did change schools so much in those formative years I did have my brother Jim, who was a year younger, and therefore pretty much my wingman all through elementary school. It would be here in Lansing, Michigan, that we would spend the next decade, and so for the first time establishing the same group of friends in school and our neighborhood was actually possible.

Junior high in the '70s was a huge leap; it was here that team school sports were first experienced, girls were something you might actually be attracted to (that is, if you could muster the courage to talk to them) and the forced integration of schools was now taking shape. Looking back, I think that is probably one of the best things that our government did at that time. School integration actually impacted us as young people, and we as teenagers had the opportunity to meet and get to know other kids of a different race. Up until that point in Michigan, schools were strictly territorial, and people were very clannish; very little integration of neighborhoods took place, so getting to know other kids from other walks of life, other races and demographics was impossible. Kids in today's world, with social networking, cellphones, texting and all of the modern diffusion of technology would have a really tough time understanding what it was like in the '70s.

I have to say one thing my parents did that finally helped me break out of my shyness shell was to make me take a speech and drama class in the eighth grade. I did not want to take this course; I had to give up woodshop for this girlie class; who in their right mind took this nonsense? Well, luckily for me, I did. It was one of those times where you are forced out of your comfort zone, you grow as a kid, and you are forced to do that really uncomfortable thing. For me it was speaking up, standing in front of a group; it was a wonderful class, and helped me tremendously. I actually was able to run for our student government at the end of the eighth grade. Junior high for us at that time was seventh through ninth, so I ran for our class vice-president position, which entailed campaigning and giving two separate speeches in front of the entire student body, running against the, what I perceived in my sense of inadequacy, really cool, popular kids. It was exciting, it was growth, and you know what? I actually won; it was a huge step toward becoming confident and liking myself.

In the '70s team sports were all we had for outside activities, so they were another way to meet people, grow friendships, and grow as a person. Frankly, it was the best part of this chapter of my life. Many of the guys I played ball with in junior and senior high are still my friends today; it's amazing how you remember these times through extracurricular activities. In our hometown I had the luxury of growing up with young men who would become outstanding college and even professional athletes; we had tremendous teams, great coaching, and learned the discipline necessary to move forward in life. I believe that the team sports, especially the junior high team sports, not only built the long-term friendships and comrades, but gave the foundation for fitness and discipline necessary to be a successful student. On a side note I believe one of the biggest failures of our public school system now is the loss of team sports at the junior high level. I think that those districts that still provide the funding and coaching, and opportunities for kids to participate in these types of activities, are going to build better students, kids, and adults as they grow up; that I am sure of.

High school was a golden time, the blending of two big junior high schools together to form one huge student body, in high school. We were Everett, home of the Vikings. Many of the boys from the other school (I was a Walter French kid; the others were mostly from Gardner junior high) I had already come into contact with through our athletics, either the school or the city league competition, so we kind of eye-balled each other when we went through that tenth grade orientation. We each thought we were better, and actually, our junior high was! We let that sense of pride disappear early though, because high school football started two weeks before school actually began, so through our dying in the summer heat with double sessions in practice we learned quickly that high school and sports was a whole different caliber; it was tough, and it was great! Being a scrub, burger-squad football player was fine with me; it was all about friendships and being on a team.

The sense of community was the key ingredient of those years; without any distraction of technology we just "grew up", grew up and partied. In the infinite wisdom of our government, and the Vietnam War, the age for legal drinking at that time in Michigan was 18. This of course meant that in high school, drinking alcohol was the norm. It was accepted, and almost encouraged. The keggers, the high school parking lot, after football game dances, disco and Motown, big hair rock, it was all part of our social dynamic, planting the seed of substance abuse and drinking that would become an issue later in life, which it did. High school in the seventies was a time for many highs, including first trying pot, and many lows.

In my junior year, 1976, my parents finally separated and later divorced; it was a very hard time. As I have said I give them both credit for a wonderful group of kids, but four boys and one girl, one income, being too young when they initially were married—I think it finally hit the breaking point, and they ended their tumultuous marriage. It was still a kind of taboo thing, this divorce thing; parents mostly still stuck it out "for the kids," which mine did for a long time. Their breakup did not help my confidence level; even though growing up until now I had made strides physically and socially, I think that seeing and living through this, especially being the oldest (at this point 16 years old), planted another seed in my mind that would take years to come to grips with. Looking back, I wonder how many other families were going through exactly the same dynamic, and it was hidden away. Probably a lot. Life goes on and you have to learn to step up and deal with things;that is the name of the game, right?

In the 1970s the world had its share of social issues, and television brought us closer to the action as that world became smaller, particularly with the advent of cable TV, which arrived in our home in the mid-seventies. The anti-war movement was huge, with the Kent State massacre occurring on May 4th, 1970. Four students were killed and nine injured, and it was all brought to our living rooms in living color through our television sets. Mandatory integration of schools was in full roar, adding anxiety to suburbia. Roe versus Wade, Watergate, the Arab oil embargo—which led to massive inflation and even a term called "stagflation"—and the worst recession in forty years, were dominant issues.

The Civil Rights movement may be identified with a primarily racial societal change; however, it also ushered in and was a springboard for women's rights. Women's rights had languished since the 1920s, but that was about to change. The National Organization of Women (NOW) was successful in 1967 in convincing President Johnson to include women in his executive orders on equal rights, specifically his Executive Order 11246, which required all entities receiving federal contracts to end discrimination in hiring. In 1969, emerging activist Bernice Sandler used the executive order to help fight for her job at the University of Maryland. Working in conjunction with NOW and the Women's Equity Action League (WEAL), Sandler filed 250 complaints against colleges and universities.

In 1970, Sandler joined Representative Edith Green's Subcommittee on Higher Education and sat in on the congressional hearings where women's rights were discussed. It was in the congressional hearings that Green and Sandler first proposed Title IX . Title IX was drafted and introduced by Congresswoman Patsy T. Mink, with the assistance of Congresswoman Green. In the hearing there was very little mention of athletics. Their focus was more specifically on the hiring and employment practices of federally financed institutions. The proposed Title IX created much buzz and gained a lot of support.

Title IX, as we know it today, was passed into law on June 23, 1972.

Title IX may not have had immediate ramifications for athletics, as it would be several years later that the scope and reach would be fully understood and implemented, however it would change the face of higher education, and in essence the whole country, as it pertains to women. Colleges, universities and the NCAA were not happy about this; radical change in higher education is difficult, but the law is the law and once the full scope was understood women gained the equal footing they deserved.

Personally, being a dad with two daughters I am glad the change took place. Girls and women have been integrated into athletics, the playing field has been leveled and opportunities now abound for children of both sexes to have the chance to compete, socialize and experience the joy of competition. Title IX was a huge and much-needed law. The '70s had many issues, some good and many not so good.

Nineteen people were killed in 1972 at the Munich Olympic Games as terrorists, known as the PLO (Palestinian Liberation Organization) attacked and murdered members of the Israeli Olympic team. Our Vice President Spiro Agnew plead no-contest to tax evasion in 1973, leaving office in shame, and then a year later, on August 8, 1974, our President Richard Nixon was impeached for the Watergate scandal, and left office. Yes, the '70s had plenty of turmoil, angst and concerns.

We had Three Mile Island, the Jonestown massacre where 900 people perished, and in 1979 the Iranian hostage crisis started as the Shah of Iran was ousted and a 444-day-long crisis began. As Iran held our citizens hostage, Penelope Laingen, wife of hostage Bruce Laingen (charge d'affaires of the embassy) tied a yellow ribbon around a tree at her home in Maryland, and a nationwide movement began. Millions of Americans also tied the yellow symbols of freedom around trees in their yards. (They stayed up until the hostages came home – more than a year later.)

On the entertainment side of this decade of change we were blessed with unbelievable content, television, film and music; the '70s was a decade of trendsetters. We had a multitude of cop shows, sitcoms and several really good family shows, and the entertainment industry was in full swing. There will probably never be another time when nicknames for television characters were "Meathead and Big Dummy" (two of my favorites).

With all of the political shifting, the morass of issues around the war and the hippies, the protests and the sorrow, we were lucky to have entertainment, something to take our minds off of a world gone off kilter.

Archie Bunker was the leader of the outrageous, and I wonder how effective his character would be in the 21st century? I can distinctly remember the first time I ever saw this sitcom; it was electric. This bigoted white middle aged man, who in today's parlance you could say "threw everyone, everything, every race, and every creed under the bus", was unbelievable. Shocking, disgraceful, outlandish "All in the Family" was the number one show for five years in a row; it was a testament to the '70s and the changes that were happening. Archie (Carroll O'Connor) and his wife Edith (Jean Stapleton) were joined by daughter Gloria (Sally Struthers) and her "Polack" husband Michael "Meathead" Stivic (Rob Reiner) as the main roles in this classic.

Now something to remember is that the advent of time shifting (recording TV shows to watch later) via the VCR was invented in 1969, but the tape was not available until 1976, which made watching your television favorites when they were initially broadcast a family event, and the norm. Diffusion of the VCR into a ubiquitous household must-have did not occur until the '80s.

Norman Lear's "All in the Family", which premiered on January 12th, 1971, then reached the milestone of five consecutive number one years, only to be supplanted in the record books by "The Cosby Show", and now "American Idol". It did not let any issue of the time go without criticism, including: racism, homosexuality, women's liberation, rape, miscarriage, abortion, breast cancer, the Vietnam War, menopause, and impotence.

Archie Bunker and his attitudes were cutting edge and his chatter brought formerly untouchable issues to mainstream television. The show was so popular that it had several spin-offs including Maude, The Jeffersons, Gloria, and a sort of reversal of "All in the Family" with the show "704 Hauser". Spinoffs from the spinoffs continued, as "Good Times" would spin from "Maude". "All in the Family" would reign supreme as number one until 1976, when another classic, "Happy Days" would take over the top spot. "All in the Family" would run from 1971 until 1979 with a total of 209 episodes.

The '70s brought many other great shows we watched as a family. Great laughs in 1972 would include NBC's answer to "All in the Family" as "Sanford and Son" premiered, starring Redd Foxx. This show and Foxx were some of my dad's favorites, and it was a direct reversal of Archie, and in my opinion much funnier; Redd Foxx was hilarious. In 2007, Time magazine included the show on their list of the "100 Best TV Shows of All Time". Humor helped our family make it through our own turbulent times, with television-mad memories, and we looked forward to our favorites, which included classics like "The Bob Newhart Show", "Happy Days", "The Love Boat", "Mork and Mindy", and of course Alan Alda and "MASH", which ran for 11 years: 1972 until 1983.

And let's not forget escapism through television, with the myriad of cop shows; there were plenty, with some of our favorites being: "Adam 12", "Kojak", "The Rockford Files" (in which James Garner was a really cool guy private detective), "The Streets of San Francisco", "Hawaii Five-O", "SWAT", "Police Women" (yes women started to become mainstream, hard to imagine) and then of course "Charlie's Angels".

1970s music was another version of escapism, and frankly it was (in my opinion) the best time for music, ever! We had the big hair rockers, like Aerosmith, Frampton, Boston, and Kiss; there was good old rock 'n roll like The Doobie Brothers, The Eagles, and Led Zeppelin; and then we had Motown classics like The Jackson Five, Stevie Wonder, Marvin Gaye, The Temptations, The Commodores, the Miracles, and the fabulous Diana Ross and the Supremes. Disco made its way into mainstream, with KC and the Sunshine Band, The Bee Gee's and—Sandy's favorite, Andy Gibb. Kool and the Gang, the Village People, Donna Summer, Earth Wind and Fire and the Spinners, and those are just a few. Acid, psychedelic, heavy metal, progressive rock, with Hendrix and Jefferson Airplane, Pink Floyd, Deep Purple and Black Sabbath; there was so many genres it was hard to keep track, but one thing was very clear, even through the fog of pot and drinking, we had some badass tunes blasting on our stereos!

Oh yeah, and we also had Farrah Fawcett in a red swimsuit emblazoned on a poster that millions had hanging on their walls... big hair, disco, cop shows and situation comedies—we needed a break from the crazy world, and people think today is tough, please!

On a side note I read this and the '60s section to my oldest daughter Ashley when she was home visiting from Wisconsin over Christmas; at that point she was 25 years old. She listened intently to my very rough draft and when I was finished, she sat there kind of stunned; kids her age have no idea, she had no idea, and this is just the highs and lows. We boomers have experienced a ton, learned, suffered and grown up. It is one of the keys to our success and I want it to become a rallying point for all of us—you see, that is totally the point, to use our vast knowledge and mentor the young'uns; they need us really badly.

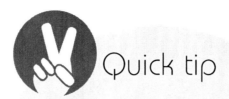

Quick tip

Ice cream headaches occur in approximately 30% of all people and are caused by eating ice cream or other cold foods in warmer weather. Researchers believe that this occurs when nerves in the roof of your mouth sense the sudden cold and the nerves signal the body to increase blood flow to the head to keep your brain warm, causing a quick-hitter headache!

9: Neurogenesis

Unlike other organs, any damage to brain cells is considered permanent and irreversible—or so it was thought. Recent research has indicated that the brain may have some capacity to regenerate and repair damaged cells. With the possibilities that stem cell research may one day offer, hope may be on the horizon for individuals suffering such crippling diseases as Huntington's, Parkinson's, and Alzheimer's disease. The ability for brain cells to regenerate themselves is known as neurogenesis.

Through the process of mitosis new cells are formed from existing brain cells. These new stem cells are born without a function. Stimulation from their physical environment causes these new cells to differentiate, or specialize, into neuronal cells. The differentiated cells migrate to different locations of the brain by means of a chemical signal. Once they move away from their origin, these cells either adapt and develop into mature neuronal cells, or they do not adapt and die. The ability of these cells to adapt to their new environment is known as plasticity.

At their final migration sites, the neuronal cells mature in the presence of chemical hormones known as neurotrophic growth factors, and acquire their lifelong functions. The new neurons become integrated into the existing synaptic circuitry. This "regenerative" development from stem cell to mature neuronal cell is the basis of neurogenesis .

It has been clearly demonstrated that our brains are much more suited to change than we ever thought possible, and that if certain "parts" fail, that others can pick up the slack. Neurogenesis is the beginning of that process.

In the 1950s and '60s the brain was metaphorically referred to as a "machine". It was believed that the brain had specialized parts for certain duties (remember the localizationist theories).

Neuroscience is on the search for the right recipe for building stronger brains as we age. Scientists know that education will help with neuron growth, and that it turns out the dendrite gyrus is very fond of exercise, which is something close to a "magic wand" for brain growth and health.

These cells are called "neuronal" because they have not matured or divided into actual neurons or glial cells. Glial cells can be referred to as support cells, and are non-neuronal cells that maintain homeostasis (balance), form myelin, and provide support and protection for the brain's neurons. In the human brain, there is roughly one glia for every neuron, with a ratio of about two neurons for every glia in the cerebral gray matter.

As the Greek name implies, glia are commonly known as the glue of the nervous system; however, this is not fully accurate. Neuroscience currently identifies four main functions of glial cells: to surround neurons and hold them in place, to supply nutrients and oxygen to neurons, to insulate one neuron from another, and to destroy pathogens and remove dead neurons. For over a century, it was believed that they did not play any role in neurotransmission. That idea is now discredited; they do modulate neurotransmission, although the mechanisms are not yet well understood .

These neuronal cells were long overlooked, because like many functions of the brain, the idea went against the "machine" theory. Remember from earlier, machine theory actually went back almost 100 years and like new ideas, the concept of the human adult brain growing new cells, "regenerating", was dismissed. It follows that science, like all academic philosophies, will not accept an idea until the empirical evidence is proven, many times over.

Until the 1980s most researchers and neuroscientists followed the philosophies of Nobel Prize winner Ramon y Cajol, who in 1913 self-assuredly wrote, "In the adult brain nervous pathways are fixed and immutable. Everything may die; nothing may be regenerated."

At the time the evidence pointed to this thought process being true; it was, however, wrong. Here I will cite and thank Dr. Norman Doidge for his work .

The evidence supporting the machine theory began to slowly unravel, when in 1965 Joseph Altman and Gopal D. Das of MIT discovered neuronal stem cells in rats. Their work was not to be believed. Then in the 1980s Fernando Nottebohm, a bird specialist, had wondered about how song birds, especially canaries, created new songs each spring. That every spring the canaries would learn a new mating tune, creating new neurons that migrated into the areas of their brains where the songs were created, added fuel to the neurogenesis scientific fire.

So, can neurogenesis strengthen mental capacity? Can non-traditional college students compete with younger, more pliable brains? Can baby boomers continue to grow new brain cells?

Dr. Rusty Gage and his team set out to understand how to encourage the creation of neuronal stem cells, and to see if it could be done. Dr. Gage and his colleague Gerd Kemperman raised mice to find out if the theory was, in fact, solid. They took aging mice, placed them in an enriched learning environment with toys, tubes, and treadmill wheels, for as short as 45 days. They then autopsied the brains of the mice, examining their hippocampi, and found a 15 percent increase in volume, and 40,000 new neurons. They also saw a 15 percent increase, compared to the mice raised without the enriched environment. In addition, they tested older mice raised in an enriched learning environment during the second half of their lives (mice normally live about two years) and found a fivefold increase in the number of neurons in the hippocampus. These mice were better at tests of learning, movement, and other events of intellect, than those raised without the enhanced environment. The test older mice developed more neurons, however not as quickly as younger mice, which in fact gave credence to the thought and empirical evidence that older subjects could in fact gain neurons.

Drs. Gage and Kemperman then discovered an ingenious way to mark brain cells with a dye called BrdU, which is absorbed into neurons at the moment they are born, and contains a marker that lights up under a microscope. The doctors asked terminally ill patients for the permission to inject them with the marker. When these patients died, Gage and Eriksson examined their brains and found new, recently formed baby neurons in their hippocampi. What an exciting finding this had to be for them—that even in dying patients, neurons continued to be born up to and all the way to the end of their lives.

Yes, in fact, a non-traditional older college student could learn; yes, in fact, baby boomers can improve cognitive skills; if the person just puts the time and effort into improving, anything is possible!

If new neurons can continue to be born, as Dr. Gage's research clearly has shown, then the potential for continued learning of new skills, growth and improvement is virtually unlimited.

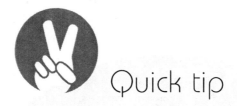 Quick tip

Cut 100 calories a day from your diet. Skip the cookies; drop the soda (just one).The cost of health care is at the heart of our nation's financial problems. If we boomers want to become the leaders of our staying-healthy movement, let's first lead by getting a firm grip on this problem. It's not going to fix itself—we have to own it! Begin by consuming fewer calories daily; just 100 calories equates to almost ten pounds in one year. Our eating habits have major consequences, which start with diabetes. Today we have approximately 28.5 million people who are diabetic, and another 66 million who are pre-diabetic; the medical bill, which is currently a paltry $174 billion a year, is expected to soar to $3.4 trillion by 2020. More than 60% of those costs are expected to be paid by the federal government. Shedding excess pounds is critical to cutting diabetes risk. So cut the 100 calories.

10: Neuroplasticity

I had the tremendous pleasure to interview Dr. Arthur Kramer on "Boomers Rock". It was not only enlightening, but really a blast. Dr. Kramer, 58 when we conducted the interview (a "sandwich boomer" like myself), is a world-renowned Professor of Psychology and Neuroscience, Director of the Beckman Institute for Advanced Science and Technology, and the Swanlund Chair. He received his Ph.D. in Cognitive/Experimental Psychology from the University of Illinois in 1984. Dr. Kramer (Art) started school at Illinois in 1979, and his research projects include topics like Cognitive Psychology, Cognitive Neuroscience, Aging, and Human Factors. A major focus of his lab's recent research is the understanding and enhancement of cognitive neural plasticity across lifespans.

Basically, Art is a badass! Oh, and did I mention stud athlete, former boxer, "don't mess with me" kind of guy? Yep, that's Art.

He is a former Associate Editor of *Perception and Psychophysics* and is currently a member of six editorial boards. Professor Kramer is also a fellow of the American Psychological Association, American Psychological Society, a former member of the executive committee of the International Society of Attention and Performance, and a recent recipient of a NIH Ten Year Merit Award.

Professor Kramer's research has been featured in a long list of print, radio and electronic media including the New York Times, Wall Street Journal, Washington Post, Chicago Tribune, CBS Evening News, Today Show, NPR and Saturday Night Live. And I am thrilled to add to that impressive list "Boomers Rock", on the all-fitness radio network, FTNS.

Dr. Kramer was kind enough to email me a couple of white papers in prep for our interview, and I want to paraphrase the definition of plasticity from the review article "Harnessing neuroplasticity for clinical applications", of which he was one of the contributing authors. It really gives a great definition of "plasticity".

"Neuroplasticity can be defined as the ability of the nervous system to respond to intrinsic or extrinsic stimuli by reorganizing its structure, function and connections."

Basically, it is the flexibility of the brain to change and adapt. Dr. Kramer told me that ten years ago this idea of the brain's ability to change was limited and fixed. That model, as he said, "is not true"; our brains can change, adapt, and improve, if we commit to behavior and actions that are positive in nature. Dr. Kramer is on the hunt, utilizing new technologies to understand how our middle-aged brains work, and his research has yielded some surprising results. Dr. Kramer and his colleagues decided to test middle-aged brains that call for split-second, swift decision making, so they went to Canada and tested air traffic controllers.

In the book *The Secret life of the Grownup Brain*[10], Barbara Strauch interviewed Dr. Kramer; they were looking for a specific model, plasticity and skills, and here is what they discovered: Apparently air traffic controllers in the U.S. are required to retire at the age of fifty-five, which in my opinion seems outrageous; however, other countries do not follow this policy and their ratio of accidents are not any higher than ours, so what gives? Are they making a mistake farming out such experienced talent? Dr. Kramer had found a group to measure, so he decided to pursue this interesting topic.

Dr. Kramer decided to visit Canada, where the policy is to allow their controllers to work until age 65. While there, Dr. Kramer ran the group of middle-aged, (older controllers), and younger controllers through a series of cognitive skills tests that were seven hours in length, and then, for a long stretch of time, had them do work that simulated their daily routine.

Dr. Kramer stated, "In real life controllers work at computers, and in our simulation we used computers and we had them do all sorts of things, just as if they were working," reported Strauch. "Sometimes they were really busy and talking to pilots and watching a screen and having aircraft coming in at different speeds. We also had them sequencing flight patterns. There were a lot of things for them to deal with."

So what was the score; what was the verdict? Amazingly, the older controllers did the same as their younger co-workers. "They clearly performed as well on simulated tasks as the younger group. There was no difference in level," stated Kramer.

Of course there are bound to be some variances; for example, in the speed in which tasks were accomplished the younger controllers scored higher. However, interestingly enough in two important cognitive areas (cognitive fluidity has been clearly linked to brain plasticity), visual orientation (imagine looking at a two-dimensional computer screen and thinking of a three-dimensional aircraft in the sky), and ambiguous differentiation (analyzing, interpreting, processing inconsistent information and developing that "gut sense"), the older controllers did just as well. As Professor Kramer states, "the thing is, if you have many years of experience, that serves you well and is very, very useful, and if an older person maintains the skills he needs, perhaps he can perform in professions that we thought he could not in the past."

So this "neuroplasticity" stuff has some serious potential, especially for the boomers, who see the next chapter, this "Indian summer of our adult lives", as an opportunity to continue to grow and give back. I think back on my grandfathers; I do remember them both very clearly—they were contradictions of their eras. One started playing golf at 50ish, becoming very good and winning tournaments, while the other was an arthritic cripple for most of his life until my grandmother died, and then at a later phase in his life had to start "doing" for himself.

Unbeknownst to both of them the adjustments and changes they made in their lives were examples of what we are now calling plasticity. In those days it was the hardwired "you get old and die" days; when the machine wears out, you retire, go sit in the living room and watch TV until you die.

"Sometimes success is due less to ability than to zeal."

—Charles Buxton

The machine metaphor of our way of thinking about our brains is being changed and rewritten. Of course certain part of our brain functionality is "pre-wired", that is, set up to function in certain fixed ways. However, what about change, what about injuries, what about health issues and illness? We now know that neurogenesis does not end until we all move on to that next place, in our spiritual place after death.

People do change continually throughout their lives; God knows I surely did. So what is the next component we need to comprehend?

Much advancement has been made in understanding these physical changes that can occur, that the machine could be rebuilt to function and potentially be improved is called "neuroplasticity".

And like the entire concept of neuroplasticity, crawling before walking, baby steps, are needed with everything. I don't care if it is fitness, weight loss, or going to college after twenty years off, our abilities are not predetermined, and that's why I am so enthralled with the pieces behind the puzzle, our tools, the modules of our brain and the power of it all. It's simply fascinating.

Granville Stanley Hall was born in 1844 in Massachusetts, and he was later to become known as the inventor of adolescence, as he became one of the leaders in the field of psychology in the U.S. He coined the term "adolescence" in 1904, in his landmark book of the same title[11], as that "middle ground of life between childhood and adulthood". I found it fascinating that Hall would become interested in life's "Indian summer" when he retired, at the age of 76!

There is so much to say about our transitional careers, the "Indian summer" of our lives. Hall wrote in the 1920s that longer lifespans, the exiting from our working lives, really had no meaning or purpose, which is a huge loss to society. Hall argued that what we indeed needed most in our society is not more youth and those youthful attitudes, but the qualities possessed by the people in the second half, Indian summer, of life. "Modern man was not meant to do his best work before forty but by is by nature, and is becoming more and more so, an afternoon and evening worker," he wrote. It is why we need to understand and grasp the functionality of our brain and its unlimited potential that can lead us into that glorious time of our lives, our perpetual Indian summer. (*"The Big Shift—Navigating the New Stage Beyond Midlife" by Marc Freedman, Public Affairs, 2011*)

Believe in your potential; the tools are there, and abilities of our incredible brain, like plasticity, make and give us unlimited potential if we work at it.

> "It's not our disadvantages or shortcomings that are ridiculous, but rather the studious way we try to hide them, and our desire to act as if they did not exist."
>
> —Giacomo Leopardi

I had become interested in the adaptability of our behavior from my own experiences with fulfilling dreams and goals, especially as it related to education and fitness several years ago when I read *The Answer* by John Assaraf and Murray Smith[12]. Even though I had questioned my own sanity in attempting college at my ripe age, I just had this feeling that it was the right thing to do, unfinished business. So in reading *The Answer*, which is actually more of a motivation and business success book, I became acquainted with Dr. Bach-y-Rita's work and neuroplasticity. Assaraf shares a story from *Discover* magazine, (Michael Abrams, "Can You See with Your Tongue?" June 1st, 2003), about a device that enabled a sixteen-year-old girl named Beth to manage to be the lead singer in her school choir, to follow her conductor perfectly, every motion and signal, maintaining a beautiful voice, and never missing a note—all while being blind.

You see, as Assaraf stated, she was wearing a device designed by the late Dr. Bach-y-Rita, a device that allowed the singer, Beth, to follow the lead of her conductor with her tongue.

Dr. Paul Bach-y-Rita, who was a founding neuroscientist at the University of Wisconsin at Madison, made his presence known; plasticity was his major field of study. He had devoted much of his career to a single, radical concept: that our senses are interchangeable. The brain, he and many other neuroscientists believe, is a body part of astonishing plasticity; if one part of it is impaired, another part can serve the same job.

As Dr. Bach-y-Rita was fond of saying, "We don't see with our eyes; we see with our brains." The ears, eyes, nose, tongue, and skin are just inputs that provide information. When the brain processes this data, we experience the five senses, but where the data come from may not be so important. "Clearly, there are connections to certain parts of the brain, but you can modify that," Bach-y-Rita stated. "You can do so much more with a sensory organ than what Mother Nature does with it."

Traditional therapy exercise routines for stroke victims end after a few weeks, when as Bach-y-Rita claimed patients "plateaued", and/or doctors lost their motivation to continue therapy. However, Bach-y-Rita knew that plateaus were temporary and part of the plasticity process; it was all part of the learning cycle, one I like to call "passionate practice".

After settling down as professor of rehabilitation medicine at the University of Wisconsin, Bach-y-Rita turned his devotion back to the senses. He knew that victims of leprosy, for instance, can lose the sense of touch in their limbs, so he developed a glove with transducers on each fingertip that were connected to five points on the forehead. When his test subjects touched something with the gloves, they felt an equal pressure on their heads. Within minutes they were able to sense the difference between rough and smooth surfaces—and they quickly forgot that their foreheads were doing the feeling.

If sight and touch can swap paths to consciousness, Bach-y-Rita reasoned, so can sound. In the 1980s, his team plugged a microphone into a vibrating belt. Low frequencies picked up by the mike tickled the left side of the waist; high frequencies tickled the right. Deaf people who donned the belt claimed it helped them read lips.

This notion dates back to 1861, when the pioneering French neurologist Paul Broca found lesions in the frontal lobe of a speechless man. Broca concluded that certain parts of the brain are responsible for certain tasks and a cascade of later research seemed to prove him right. Most recently, functional MRI and PET scans (remember earlier descriptions) have shown that different areas of the brain light up depending on whether a person is identifying colors, recognizing faces, registering emotions, or learning a language.

What we do changes our brains, the architecture, the wiring, and the mapping, which is now why Dr. Bach-y-Rita's work is so influential, why it is imperative for everyone—but especially boomers—to grasp the fact that our wiring is "plastic", our brains and lives are not "fixed", and that what we do with our lives determines the health of our bodies and brains.

Experiments have shown that those animals and humans that live in an enriched and stimulating environment (for test animals like mice rats, that would be toys in their cages), will tend to have healthy and better functioning bodies, with better-developed brains and more connections, and are happier and live longer. In humans there is ample evidence that suggests the brain continues to progress in response to external stimuli, that the development of our brains, the mapping and expansion of our positive outlooks and behaviors, is linked directly to plasticity.

It's getting back to the old saying, "Use it or lose it!"

Studies have shown, for example in 1994 in the *Journal of the American Medical Association*, that those people with fewer than eight years of education were twice as likely to become demented, and those who had lower education and lower-level occupations were three times as likely.

Children both grow and prune back synaptic connections at a furious rate as they develop, but the process all but stops in adulthood. Many researchers still believe, therefore, that a damaged brain causes permanent deficits.

Grow and prune, prune and grow; the process never stops. It is where the "use it or lose it" philosophy is so important; we are what we do and we do what we believe, so does that make sense?

Neurons release neurotransmitters that are taken up by specific receptors, but many glial cells (Remember the support cells, glia; keep these in mind because we are going to talk about support cells very soon; just think "myelin") receive and emit neurotransmitters that float through the brain as free agents. Some glial cells congregate near lesions, for instance, and in areas of the brain where learning is going on.

You see how this wiring system keeps popping up?

Dr. Michael Merzenich has been touted as "the world's leading researcher on brain plasticity" by Irish neuroscientist Ian Robertson. Dr. Merzenich is THE MAN when it comes to the topic of brain plasticity.

In his early sixties, he holds more than fifty patents, is a member of the prestigious National Academy of Sciences, who nearly thirty years ago showed how a monkey brain could reassemble itself, and is now a Professor emeritus at the University of California at San Francisco, and one of the founders of the elite Posit Science. Dr. Merzenich is the Superman of plasticity research and development.

Say that paragraph three times fast; Dr. M. really is the man.

Dr. Merzenich is insistent that the older brain (listen up, Boomers!), can be trained to be much more efficient if we only practiced at it harder.

Early in his career, Dr. Merzenvich developed with his team the most commonly used design for the cochlear implant, which allows congenitally deaf children to hear. His current work regarding plasticity involves the way learning-disabled people improve their cognitive skillsets and perception. This work, and his series of plasticity-based computer programs (namely "Fast For-Word"), have enabled thousands to improve their cognitive skillsets, through plasticity and change. Fast For-Ward is disguised as a children's game and has helped people with a lifetime of learning and cognitive deficiencies, sometimes in only 30 to 60 hours of treatment. Our cerebral cortex (the thin layer of our outer brain), Merzenich says, "is actually selectively refining its processing capacities to fit each task at hand; it is learning how to learn." (*"The Brain That Changes Itself"*, *Norman Doidge M.D. Viking Press, 2007)*

Merzenich was not on a quest to comprehend how the brain changes. He actually stumbled upon the comprehension of the brain's ability to reorganize its routes, the maps. And he was not the first and only neuroscientist to demonstrate neuroplasticity; however, it was his experiments, which were conducted early in his career, that started the seismic shift in the neuroscience world away from the fixed "machine model" to a more "plastic" moldable brain model. It was through these early experiments that he showed how our brain mapping changes depending on what we do over the course of our lives.

Encore lives, Indian summer potential – Boomers, we have a lot to do and the potential for great achievements are at our own disposal; head moving in the right direction—are you catching my drift here?

Back to the college story:

And let me make something clear to you—it is fully my intention to encourage anyone and everyone about going back to school; I do not consider myself as anything special. To be perfectly frank and honest I considered myself kind of a loser in a way, because I was a dropout and then a non-traditional. But goals and dreams take precedence over anything else. I will cover in detail behavior and all of that later; I kind of figured that we needed to get the physical side of this first and then the conscious versus non-conscious in its own section. I hope you agree.

Anyway, I talked about that first class, and all four hundred college students, the professor and all that. What is really important to understand is the function that is happening behind the scenes, which this neurogenesis, plasticity thing is really happening and it is what is so exciting about the whole deal. It really is a "use it or lose it" mindset that we have to completely believe in. We all have the potential, and these key brain activities can and will occur for anyone. Hey, if it did for me it most certainly can for you.

When you start a long process of learning, remember that when we were in school as youngsters and teenagers we all had twelve years to build the foundation. So it will take time, and every class and every person's experience will differ. The first few classes were not so great; to be honest, they sucked, but the thing that kept me going was the dream and being stubborn. I knew I blew it when I was younger, no doubt; however, at forty years old I looked at it in a completely different light. I wanted it, really badly. And I appreciated the chance; before it was not like that, not at all. Younger people do not see the value in higher education, but Boomers—we do!

So as my neurogenesis and plasticity continued to improve, we move forward. Let me give you some advice right now though, especially those of you who have not started back yet, take all the advice you receive about classes with a grain of salt, and go ahead and listen, because people will give you unsolicited advice—some good, some not so. The thing I want you to know about my time was this, someone's easy cake walk just might be your nightmare. It definitely happened to me, many times, and you know what happens is you lull yourself into this false sense of security, so beware. All classes take time and effort, and you will probably find some that work out better than others, so never let your guard down and whatever you do, start strong and don't get behind. Stress does not help plasticity; in fact, I think it stops the new brain map from forming and that, my friends, is bad.

Remember to go to office hours. Some of the best learning, neurogenesis and brain mapping happen while you talk to a teacher or professor, meet them, tell them your story and befriend them. You will thank me for that. And you will be amazed at how much you learn; it really is crazy. You know what is crazier yet? Traditional students don't really go to office hours, hardly ever. Ask any professor, and they will tell you it does not happen, so use that to your advantage. Socialization and learning are huge. Continuing education is even huger!

My doctor friends, including Dr. Bartzokis, have said that nothing speeds brain atrophy more than being immobilized in the same environment. This is something I think that boomers have become accustomed to; we coast along in our habits, and that reduces our brain mapping. Think about this: monotony undermines our dopamine (that's the pleasure chemical in our brain), and attention systems crucial to maintaining brain plasticity. In addition, a cognitively rich physical activity such as learning new dances will probably help ward off balance problems and have the added benefit of being social, which also preserves brain health. Studies have been done that suggest that individuals with more education seem better prepared for mental decline. The theories suggest that those times spent learning, academically and or physically, can build a "cognitive fallback" of more developed networks in your brain, through plasticity and neurogenesis, which can be used as we age.

11: Myelin

As Alexander Graham Bell continued to build out the telephone network it was always the wire that made the difference in the quality of service. Since the beginning people were just amazed that this newfangled invention could actually work, and just like in the 21st century with personal computers and handheld devices and cellular networks, as we become accustomed to this QOL we take it for granted. However, for a long time it was party lines and crank phones; the network and its abilities were very limited. Making a long distance phone call, up until the 1970s, was still a big deal and it was costly. The network and the brain (central office equipment) were the backbone, the central nervous system and brain of the world communication system. Similar to the human brain, understanding potential and technology held the key to change and rapid growth.

At this point we have two of the three components of the human communication system, which is the backbone, the "central office": neurogenesis, our ability to continually our entire lives give birth to new neurons, resupplying our brain with fresh tools; and neuroplasticity, the ability to take external stimuli and—with work—remap, learn, and create new pathways with unlimited potential. And now comes the heavy lifter of the bunch, myelin.

It was the reading of Daniel Coyle's *The Talent Code*[13] that started the whole topic of myelin in my mind. It was the catalyst for building my energy to learn more; I was fascinated. I did contact Dan and interviewed him on "Boomers Rock", and I asked him point blank, "WHY THIS?" Dan has always been interested in performance, the "how" behind the "who", so to speak, and he really did not know much about the subject of myelin. He soon discovered that in all of his travels researching these talent hotbeds, several key things kept occurring and the evidence started to stack up; this myelin stuff is big, so what exactly is it?

Remember earlier when we discussed the advent of MRI and the tools to see inside one's brain, the PET scans and the glowing neurons. Those tools also allow a neuroscientist, like Dr. George Bartzokis of UCLA, to start answering questions on this "white matter". This white matter is made up of myelin, which is the fatty outer coating of the trillions of nerve fibers that make up our central and peripheral nervous system; it is the insulator. The insulator, much like telephone wire's plastic sheathing, protects the electrical signal from degrading as it passes through the network on its way to our central office, the brain. The better the insulator, the clearer the signal and the faster the transmission, the better response and action; it is not magic, it is myelin. As Dr. Bartzokis mentioned during our interviews, "What do good athletes do when they train? They send precise impulses along wires that give the signal to myelinate that wire. They end up, after all the training, with super-duper wire-lots of bandwidth, a high speed T-3 line. That's what makes them different than the rest of us." BOOM, I was hooked. T-3 line, bandwidth, wire, throughput, I get it. Myelinated nerves are like the difference in the first undersea telephone cable in the 1900s and fiber optic cable now. This is huge, and now I get it. Talking to Dr. Bartzokis was like going to office hours in college: it was great!

Dr. George Bartzokis, M.D. is Professor in the Department of Psychiatry at the David Geffen School of Medicine at UCLA and has been doing brain research for over twenty years. Dr. Bartzokis uses magnetic resonance imaging (MRI) of the brain to assess development and degeneration, and the relationship of these processes to disease development (such as schizophrenia, bipolar disorder, and substance abuse) as well as degeneration (such as Alzheimer's disease and fronto-temporal dementia).

Dr. George, (Bartzokis) has developed a novel conceptualization of the human brain that focuses on myelin. Myelin is the "insulation" of the wires (nerves) that makes up what he likes to say is our brain's "amazing Internet". This myelin-focused model of the brain proposes that the development, maintenance, and degeneration of myelin are central to acquiring our cognitive and behavioral abilities, as well as our vulnerability to many common diseases that plague our species across our lifespans. He has also developed several novel magnetic resonance imaging (MRI) techniques to measure brain myelin. His research aims to use MRI measures to better define healthy brain characteristics and identify abnormalities at very early stages when treatment interventions may slow, stop, and possibly reverse progression of such diseases.

So you think achy joints are the primary reason we slow down as we age? Think again. Everything begins with the brain, and at age 40 (or so) our decline could already be starting. How fast we can throw a ball or run down a basketball court depends on many things, but primarily it's our brain's ability to fire signals, our nerves' ability to deliver those signals to our muscles, and it is myelin that helps the signal get to the intended destination, on time and in sequence.

Think fiber optic cable versus the first leaky undersea telephone cable. Catch my drift here?

So for boomers thinking along the myelin line it is no wonder that people look back on the younger days and wistfully think about regaining youth. Could it be the myelin that we really desire to recapture? Looking back on younger days is natural; you always reminisce about the days of ample energy, unconfined exuberance, that attitude of invincibility, when our myelin was in full growth.

Think about the advancement of medical imaging that we spoke of earlier; it has really been less than fifteen years that neuroscientists like Dr. George (Bartzokis) have really had the tools to unravel the white matter, and it is lucky for us that he has. Myelin is "revolutionary" according to him. It is the key to talking, walking, reading, playing the piano (or for me it is going to be learning to play the drums. . .bucket list, digress, onward). *It is the being human.*

While Dr. George does not disregard the topics of neurogenesis or plasticity, it is his opinion that the neuroview needs some tweaking. Think about these three simple facts:

- Human movement, thoughts, and feelings are finely tuned electrical signals sent from our nervous systems (peripheral and central) through the interconnection of neurons and synapses, then returning back, constantly firing, supercomputer processing. Think again Internet, fiber optic cable, Google search, only hundreds of times faster. Get it?

- Myelin is the protective insulation of our fiber optic cable, nerves, which allow this electrical signal to quickly communicate, reach out to its intended receptor site, delivering that message to the right place at the right time.

- The more we fire the signals, the more myelin grows, and wraps, and wraps and grows. It is optimization at its finest, and it is why passionate practice (more on that shortly) is so critical to success, in everything we do. Grandma and mom always said practice makes perfect. Guess what? In the world of neuroscience, they were right all along.

"What do good athletes do when they train?" Dr. George stated, "They send precise impulses along wires that give signals to myelinate that wire." Skill is myelin protection that wraps neural circuits and that grows according to certain signals. The story of ability and aptitude is the story of myelin.

Brain insight lesson one: neurogenesis, plasticity and myelination are the end results of electrical impulses sent through our bodies' electrical networks. Our brains consist of 100 billion or so neurons, interconnected by synapses. Each conscious and non-conscious movement, behavior, attitude, thought—everything starts here. We see it, we experience it, we love it, and we do it, whatever it is—it is processed and mapped and stored.

Brain insight lesson two: the more we do the same behaviors, develop that route, the circuit, the deeper it is mapped, and the more automatic it will become. The more we stash things into the subconscious the more automatic it becomes. Automaticity, building of habits, muscle memory (think riding a bike, or robot-driving to work) that ability to develop the innate skill is the puzzling recipe; we work at building the skill (passionate practice) and get so good at it we forget we even learned it in the first place—myelination at its best.

Okay, so we continue to build out the telephone network, and long distance phone calls; we are almost to the satellite age and in the 1950s cable television come along. Originally it was designed to help promote the over-the-air television signals (think analog) in outlying areas of Pennsylvania; lots of hills cause transmission issues. So the cable network was born, the telephone network continues to improve, and computers... well, they are just around the corner but for us boomers it was a great time to be born and be a kid; the times they were a'changing. It is all about the network. Cable TV was a great idea but the really great idea was the wire, coaxial cable; you know the black stuff we now take for granted? It is called throughput, the ability to pump a lot of information electrically speaking, think bits and bytes, down a conduit. Just like our nervous system, great wire, and great content, equal great transmission. Color TV—you see where I am going with this? Great insulation provides the environment for fast, super-fast, robust transmission; myelin is insulation and it does the exact same thing.

Myelin has the ability to take a small pathway and build the insulation around it and create a lightning-fast super expressway. The signals, the impulses that would just lumber along, now speed up and merge into the carpool lane; it is the Autobahn—it is called the refractory period, the time when a cell is capable of receiving another stimulus, and myelin helps to shorten that time. Myelin has the ability to regulate the overall speed, because like a great concert, you must have the timing down to make the orchestra sound perfect.

It happens like this, the supporter cells are called oligodendrocytes and astrocytes; they sense nerves firing, and like an automatic cable sheathing machine wrap myelin around the firing nerves. The more they fire the faster the wrapping, the thicker the myelin the faster the transmission, and on and on, get it? In the world of telephony or data transmission it is called attenuation and throughput. Dr. George uses bandwidth as his metaphor; I hope you see the pattern, because it really is the same thing. It is one of the reasons I was so drawn to this topic in the first place; there really are so many similarities between the 21st century data networks and our bodies' fitness and myelin.

The key is timing, like in a packet-switched internet world. Packet loss is bad—think YouTube and sound and picture goofiness; not good. Signals have to travel at the precise speed, arrive at the correct time, and myelination is the brain's way of controlling speed.

We all have the ability to build our skill circuits, our routes, our internal network -of wiring, which is what is so exciting about putting it all together—the possibilities. Now that we understand the concept, the physiological side of myelin and what it means to our brain, then the next step to improving, to getting better, is simple, and it is called practice!

12: Passionate practice

In my reading, learning and interviewing I saw several different descriptions of "practice". Mass practice, hard practice, dedicated practice, deep practice; didn't Mom always say "practice makes perfect"? Guess what—she was right all along.

Perfect practice, practical practice, timely practice, focused practice, long practice. I like this one: "Passionate Practice". They are all good. No, they are all great, but I still like mine the best—passionate practice.

I guess Mom was right. Because of the inherent nature of our brains' plasticity, practice holds the key to everything. Without practice, we don't have mapping, and without mapping we do not have plasticity, and without the firing and coordination of it all we don't have myelination, so it really is true—Mom was right. Practice does make perfect, and it is not easy... not in the least, but again with the metaphor, anything worth having is worth working for. Passion is where it is at; it is all about how bad you really want it. Incrementally achieving your goals, baby steps, increasing difficulty, firing, firing and more firing of circuits, is the only way.

How did Michael Jordan become so great, or Earvin "Magic" Johnson, or Jack Nicklaus, or Beethoven, or Mozart, or Bill Gates? Hard work, that's how. It was a passion for success and an intense desire to improve—nothing special, just effort and, of course, PRACTICE! Healthy habits known to boost brain activity:

1. Walk and talk

2. Vary routine

3. Get smart

4. Play

5. De-stress

6. Sleep

7. Imagine

8. Party

9. Eat right

10. Know your numbers

Cognitive learning is an ongoing life skill dependent upon the individual's motivation—it takes daily training and practice, and let's talk about 10,000 hours. This is where things get really interesting.

> "If a man is called to be a street-sweeper, he should sweep streets even as Michelangelo painted, or Beethoven composed music or Shakespeare wrote poetry. He should sweep streets so well that all the hosts of heaven and earth will pause to say, here lived a great street-sweeper who did his job well.
>
> ~Martin Luther King Jr.

13: 10,000 hours or ten years

10,000 hours. That seems like a lot, and it is; however, it is the hard work and passionate practice that pay off in the end. In Malcolm Gladwell's book *Outliers*[14], I was first introduced to the concept of this "10,000 hour rule". Yes, it takes time to get better, and it all depends on how badly you want your goal as to how really good you can become. The 10,000 hours came up over and over; it really was kind of amazing, but before we get into that check this out first:

What Gladwell developed in *Outliers* was this profound story of successful people, brainpower and ambition; the major "how" we reach that pinnacle. He took a different tack, looking around success, beside those who were outstanding and putting together an interesting body of work. I like to think of this as the mixing of all of our physiological brain powers, neurogenesis, plasticity and myelin, (especially myelin), and combining the hard work attitude of "anything is possible" mindset, if you please. That and some external factors such as when people are born, are a launching pad to greatness.

Gladwell did some research on young hockey players and he discovered that there was an interesting clue into greatness on the ice: when they were born, specifically what month of the year. Now you may ask why this is relevant, and what does this have to do with baby boomers, success and so forth; just hear me out. Gladwell's detective work determined that young future players of success were born at certain times of the year, specifically early January through August, and that being just a little bit older gave these kids their first slight advantage, a small amount of size difference and an edge, just enough to give them a leg up. And it is not only in athletics but in academia also, as the slightly older children scored better on tests. The age difference can lock a child into an achievement pattern that can be positive and/or negative.

Growing up, I had this same thing happen to me; it was little league baseball. I was born on May 30th, and the cutoff date for baseball was June 1st, so by my being born two days before the cutoff date I missed playing in the lower division for an additional year. That could have meant an extra year where I was a bigger and more experienced player, playing more, getting more playing time and developing, which at that age is a huge advantage. I realized it growing up so when I read Gladwell's stats on the hockey player the memory was right there in my synapse: been there, done that!

So understanding this thought, we can move forward with my original point, which is, perhaps success is not a born into a genius- or savant-like mechanism, and possibly if we look at the factors that are built into success we can replicate the process, build greatness, learn and master a skill, remap our brains and make ourselves better, and develop the myelin through passionate practice!

Boomers beware, there is potential greatness in all of us; we just need to work at it. Check this out—a guy named Bill Joy.

In *Outliers, ("Outliers", Malcolm Gladwell, Little Brown and Company 2008)*, Gladwell introduces the reader to what he described as a "gawky teenager" who was a student at the University of Michigan the year the state-of-the-art computer center opened in 1971, a 16-year-old "Most Studious Student" from his high school (not far from where I write this) at North Farmington High School, which as Gladwell put it, "a no-date nerd." Joy reportedly was thinking about becoming a mathematician or scientist or something along those lines when he stumbled across the new computer center late in his freshman year, and became "hooked." And that is what it takes to become great. Love and fire of the skillset, the sport, the music, whatever, a combination of luck and drive—it is not just a gift; you have to earn it through effort. It takes understanding all of this for the picture to become clear, and that's where the 10,000 hours come into play.

You can read the details of Bill Joy on many different sites, how he grew into and worked his way into greatness, becoming one of the key players in the computer revolution, a founder of Sun Microsystems, and a key player and code writer for the backbone of many systems on the internet to this day, some 25-plus years later. He earned it, he worked it, he put in his 10,000 hours, and of course he was indeed talented, but the bottom line is he worked at it, period!

K. Anders Ericsson: 10 years and/or 10,000 hours

In the 1990s psychologist K. Anders Ericsson and two associates came up with a study to help make this 10,000-hour argument more concrete. His associates from the Berlin Academy of Music divided the school's violinists into three groups. In the first group there were the "stars", the students with the talent to become world class. In their second group they placed the students who were judged to be "good", and the third group they categorized as never to play professionally, and were destined to become public school music teachers. All of the students were asked the same question in the survey, which was, "Over the course of your entire career, ever since you picked up the violin, how many hours have you practiced?" All of the students reportedly had started playing at approximately the same age, around five, and in the first few years the time spent practicing was very similar, about two to three hours a week. This, however, changed when the children reached the age of eight.

Around this time the "star" pupils began a journey of advanced, passionate practice, practicing more than six hours a week at first by age nine, eight hours a week by age 12, 16 hours a week by age 14, more and more, until the age of around 20 they were hammering home, with a purpose, over 30 hours a week, with the true commitment of improvement and diligence. By the time it was all said and done, they had accumulated over 10,000 hours of practice, reaching elite status, while the good students had averaged 8,000 hours and the future music teachers had averaged merely 4,000 hours. The compelling fact was that Ericsson and his colleagues could not find any "naturals" in any of the students; it was the dedicated effort and work that set them apart, the ability to passionately practice.

Ericsson, along with his colleagues in his field of Psychology, established a notable body of work, documented in several books, most recently in the *Cambridge Handbook of Expertise and Expert Performance*. It has a central, overarching theme that every expert in any field is the product of ten thousand hours of passionate practice. Ericsson termed it "deliberate practice", which he characterized as working on technique, seeking constant serious advice, which in turn would add a learning component to the process. Mom's "practice makes perfect" fits well here.

As Dan Coyle intimated in *Talent Code, ("The Talent Code", Daniel Coyle, Bantom, 2009)*, Ericsson, along with Bill Chase and Herbert Simon, researchers who with Ericsson worked through this, which validated the "Ten-year Rule", which was an intriguing finding, dating back to the early 19th century. So, what about the genius, the mystical know-it-all protégé? Many objections were encountered, which Ericsson coolly explained by referring to Dr. Michael Howe of Exeter University in his book *Genius Explained*: "Even Mozart was estimated to have completed 3,500 hours of practice with his instructor father by the age of six. Yes it was an almost obsessive desire to practice that makes the difference, passion at its foremost, but it explains plenty." And as Ericsson stated, "there's no cell type that geniuses have that the rest of us don't"; it really is about the quantity and quality of the work—that's the bottom line.

14: The '80s— Southern California and the lost decade

Having graduated from high school in 1977, and being that we, as a family were now a single-parent household with five children, I had to attend the local community college when that time arrived. In the beginning of college I was a "know-everything" little turd; I thought I was really big stuff, living in the basement of my mom's home, being the "Man" of the house, but I was totally clueless. At that point in the world many of my friends did not go on to higher education; they went directly into the auto industry, being that we had a huge Oldsmobile plant in our hometown, and at that time things were really good with autos, with high pay, great sales; it was all good. So I spent part of my time going to school, doing pretty well, and hanging out in the basement smoking weed. I just figured that there was no way all of that smoke would wind up in the rest of the house where my brothers and sister and mom lived; no way. You see what I mean about being clueless. My mom finally asked me to stop smoking in the basement, and me with all of my worldliness said, "No, I would just as soon move out," so I did... kinda.

For the next month I bummed around town staying at friends' houses, girlfriend's house, any house that would put me up; I was going to show my mom I was a big boy and could take care of myself. Well, jobless college students don't have a huge list of friends to sponge off of and pretty soon it was reality-check time—I had to get a job and find some place to live. This would be the first of many mistakes, or a life lesson of the late '70s for this new grownup.

I did find a job, I did get some room-mates and I did re-enter college, and through the next two years learned the hard ways of part-time student, full-time work, and it basically sucked. I lucked out and scored a great job as a weekend warrior at the auto plant; you had to be a full-time student, which luckily at that point I was again. I made some great money for the little bit of work I did, and I got my two years of school done. The summer before I had been asked to work full-time in the plant (and let me tell you once you work seven days a week in a motor plant, in production work, on the afternoon shift, you make some money), but you come to appreciate what college could do for you. I admire the guys who put up with that lifestyle, but that work sucked so bad I never wanted to do that full-time, ever! I was ready to head to a real University, living in a dorm and getting the degree I now had a much better idea I wanted. I have a real empathy for any and all production workers, and those my age who stuck it out, I want you to know, read this book and learn, because that time was rough for me, but I can't imagine how bad it was for you.

My dream of the University (Western Michigan) was about to be put on hold—for good, it would turn out.

The spring of 1980 I had the opportunity to relocate to Southern California, through just dumb luck and my sister spending some time there, so I made the decision to go for it.

I had always dreamed of living in the Golden State, I had looked at the college catalogs while attending the community college, and if I got a chance I was there; this was my chance, so I took it, with two of my buddies. It was road trip time—this little adventure would last 15 years and I would not move back to my home state of Michigan until 1995.

I could justify this move because, at that time, California had the best state-supported University system in the country. I mean, where else could you go to school, with six or more credits for under $200 a semester? No where. Not to mention the unemployment rate in Michigan at that time, due to the oil embargo of the '70s, was almost 14% in 1980 and would peak at almost 16% by 1983; there was no future here.

So off to So-Cal it was. In April of 1980, I pulled the trigger and landed in Orange County, California, Anaheim to be exact—home of Disneyland and Knott's Berry Farm, the beaches and the freeways. I thought I had landed in paradise; that, in itself, was truly a paradox. One month later, May 30, 1980, I sat in an apartment with my two Michigan roommates, Tim Dunham and Craig Bowersox, a couple of new friends and neighbors in our one-bedroom apartment and celebrated my 21st birthday. Beer, Yukon Jack, marijuana and cocaine— it's amazing I can even remember the sordid details but this was, unbeknownst to me, the pattern of behavior that would revolve in my life for the next 15 years; a rollercoaster of activities that consumed my life.

So-Cal, the '80s and partying; look out because here came the lost decade.

To take advantage of the educational benefits of the California State University system you had to be a resident for one year. I figured that was perfect to get acclimated and adjust to the new lifestyle, make friends, and find all of the benefits of North Orange County in the 1980s. I had no idea that the entire world was changing, that drug use and drinking were the acceptable, almost completely encouraged behavior. Hey, for a guy who had been trying to discover himself, what better way to do it than through destructive behavior? Everyone was doing it, and like the sheep I was, I was happy to follow along. Having a mandatory year to establish myself, it was time to find a job, any job, so time to hit the streets and get busy. Luckily for me (in a way I always had the mindset of being the luckiest guy around), jobs were quite plentiful at this juncture in history, and even though I did not own a car, and living in southern California with no wheels is almost an impossibility, I found a job in a tool warehouse, got my roommate a job there, and made enough friends so that carpooling was easy. So here we were the first summer: job, an apartment, sand volleyball court at our apartment, pool, new friends, and party central; it could not have been any better. However, this was planting the seeds for my future problems with drug and alcohol abuse, but at this point who cared? We were indestructible and living in the moment, working, partying, sunshine and So-Cal. I had arrived.

So I stuck to the plan and actually picked up a class at the local JC, Fullerton to be exact; all they required was a driver's license as proof of residency. As the nomads of young guys we wound up in a house in a swanky residential neighborhood, and I was accepted to the University, California State University Fullerton, where I decided to become a full-time student again, borrow money through student loans, and live with a part-time job with my friends in the swanky frat house. Through the University I landed a part-time job at a bowling center right next to campus—perfect, close. I had bought a beater car so my commute was nothing, everything was great; however, problems with this situation were brewing. Did it have anything to do with my newfound passion for hard partying? Of course, the descent into the dark abyss was clearly taking place. Obsessive-compulsiveness does not work well with cocaine, marijuana and booze.

The job I had picked up at the bowling center evolved into a career. Everyone liked the new kid; I was what they called a "porter", a fancy name for janitor. I was amazed at how much they liked my work—I mean, the Michigan college kid; I was actually shocked. The job was easy, and I quickly advanced, right into bar tending; can you see the handwriting on the wall? I had found my niche, my place, and I blossomed into the lead guy. Hey, to run a bar you need only a few skills: personality, know some people, and make it accommodating to a party; perfect, I was the man. In one year I took a bar making around 6-7 grand a month up to 30; I was a rock star in my owner's and manager's eyes, and the money—well, let's just say here I am 22-23 years old. Who needed college? I was on the fast track to living large, and I did; it was such a blur. Screw taking classes; I was sucking anyway. I had lost my edge, all of the importance of education and the future. Who cared? It was all about the now! It all fed into my behavioral issues, and just like for many other twenty-somethings in the early '80s, partying was the encouraged and accepted norm. It was work at night, play golf during the day, eat like crap, drink like a fish, smoke weed like a factory and snort coke like an elephant. Someday I would find out you have to become accountable; however, that was the furthest thing from my mind.

Here is an example of just one of the many road trips that could have led to me or any of my friends dying, through the excessiveness of the bar life. Actually this was me coming out of a situation where I should have never made it. God was looking out for my stupid ass. Check this out—true story:

I had worked a Saturday night tending, so for once I was still sober and we had a road trip planned to go to the famous Colorado River. Now I had heard the stories about this "river" in the desert. The Colorado River is the state line between California and Arizona, so we headed out after I closed the bar at three in the morning. Starting a road trip at that time of the day, or night, or whatever it was, is not a good start, and especially since my roomies had all been partying (what else is new?) I finally convinced my buddy, (who was driving and weaving all over the road, falling asleep) that maybe I should drive; he finally let me after several near misses. We traded seats on the side of the 10 freeway, in the middle of the desert, and as I started to drive he decided to take the T-top off of his side of the car, while it was moving; not a good idea. The thing flew off, smashed into a million pieces and was an omen of the whole weekend. We did arrive at this Godforsaken place; it was a dump, but I was so exhausted I did not care. I needed to sleep so I could party later.

Where we camped, I guess you could call it "camped"— it was not Midwest camping by any stretch, was basically the desert, and this portion of the Colorado River, this fast-moving ditch of water no more than fifty feet wide, was not at all what I envisioned as this great spot. Basically I was not impressed, at all. Now let's be fair and clear, I have seen pictures of some outstanding spots, Lake Havasu, Lake Mead, all are derived from this ditch of water so I mention this to give equal billing, anyway. We were here for two reasons: to ride off-road three-wheelers (this is the time before they were outlawed for being unsafe) and to party. Learning to ride an ATV three-wheeler is pretty straightforward, and we spent the bulk of the day doing just that—no helmets, flip flops and drinking, a great combination. The real fun begins when the sun goes down; for the experienced people, those who actually own these toys and have done this stuff, riding around at night for them is old news, but for us Midwest party boys it was time to fly around in the desert by the moonlit desert; it was exhilarating, and we did this for most of the night. That was until I decided I was going to lead the pack. There must have been eight or ten of us on these man-killers; it was late, like three in the morning, and we had been going hard at it all night. It's amazing what youthful twenty-something energy, a bunch of cocaine, and plenty of Jack Daniels and beer can do for your energy level, and confidence, and stupidity. It was a perfect blend for something really bad to happen, and it did. As I said I had taken the lead on this excursion. Doing 25 to 35 doesn't sound like much; however, in the pitch dark of the California / Arizona desert it is cooking. This is the wilderness and the desert is not forgiving. Being a one-day riding expert leading this tribe I went straight on this trail, but unbeknownst to me it was a turn. I launched myself into a dry washout of a flash flood river, which is very common in the desert, and you would clearly see this during the day, but it was about 20 feet deep and I was airborne! God has mercy on the stupid and the drunken fools because somehow my natural instinct was to let go of the trike, and tuck and roll. As the three wheeler smashed into the river-bed, completely totaling it, I landed in a perfect roll and somehow did not die. That's not to say I was unhurt; that would have been impossible. I was all beat up, but apparently through the Almighty's wisdom I was spared death, only to live through severe gashes and contusions. The Lord protects drunken fools. We headed back to our campsite, or whatever you would call sleeping in the desert open air, slamming down Jack Daniels to numb the pain of the stupidity that had just occurred. Maybe it helped; I lived.

The next morning I woke up to the sound of people talking about the three-wheeler that they had hauled up from a dry river bed completely destroyed; those things are really tough, and it takes a lot to break them. I heard the people commenting on how hard it is to break these things, and did the guy who was on it live? At that point I woke up to assess my wounds. No broken bones, no dislocated joints, which for me having shoulder issues is a miracle in itself, just deep holes in my skin, my back, shoulder, foot, legs all scraped and deep contusions; I would live although it was going to be a long recovery. That was my first and last experience in desert off-road ATV riding.

That story is just one of many California living experiences; I have thought about writing a memoir on just this part of my life... maybe someday. The point being, and what I am trying to paint the picture of, is the whole decade of the '80s had this type of behavior. The "I am Spartacus" indestructible dude mentality, this was my lost decade; this is where the behavior of abuse started to become deeper and deeper; it was a long process and we called it having fun. I am sure many of us have very similar histories of overindulgence, stories and histories. It is why I cannot remember many of the concerts and ballgames, parties and bar-b-ques; they all run together as a montage of haze and excess. These were not mistakes; they were poor decisions that helped me to become what I am today. With that the realization that drug use and alcohol abuse is not the way to live the life that I want; that I value the little things, that doing these things, living through it all has become my blessing to share with others, the ability to change and come out of the dark abyss of dependency.

I did have a failed marriage during this time. It is no wonder; we were two people who were users and abusers, who were destined for failure. It fed into my insecurities of failed relationships, reminding me of my parents and their long-term dislike for each other. It gave me the perfect excuse to feed my codependent destructive behaviors, abusive substance use, and wasteful financial decisions. And I witnessed the L.A. Riots first-hand, up close and personal as I drove down an empty Hollywood freeway the second day of the riots, trying to get home from a job in the San Fernando Valley. To say the sight of L.A. burning is scary would be a huge understatement.

However, it was not all a huge negative; there were many positives, hard as it is to believe. That is where the eternal optimist will always see the light of goodness, that learning from mistakes, growing to value your life, and the good people who are in it.

I am blessed to have had those times; they taught me to value the preciousness of what is good. My oldest daughter was a gift from God, born in 1986. Ashley, though raised in a dysfunctional setting as a young child, still had love heaped on her, and she now has heard me talk about my poor judgments as a young adult, teaching her not to make the mistakes that were the encouraged behaviors of the 1980s. She has grown into a very successful young woman with a bright future.

The long-term friendships I still possess with my California friends are near and dear to me. The professional education and business experience was invaluable. The life lessons, good and bad, make me appreciate my life and sobriety now. You can pull many positives from this time; however, the bottom line is this: the accountability of poor behaviors will always be mine, and the understanding that living that quality of life doesn't happen through chemical adoration; dependency is a dark road—I know; I walked it. Don't let the past get in the way of the future; take it and grow, teach and become better. Do not dwell on past poor decisions. They are over; they are done. Life is like that great tree that weathers the storm, loses limbs and branches in inclement weather, only to sprout anew and continue to grow, bigger and stronger for the wear.

There is so much yet to come; through adversity grows opportunity! Our bodies and minds are miraculous gifts, which can change and improve; yes, through adversity, opportunity grows.

Thank you God for the gift of change and improvement, learning and wisdom, making a promise to give back, I owe my life to my guardian angel.

Remarkably, life is such a wonderful ride and journey. Take each day and count your blessings; I do!

Content would continue to be king in the 1980s; the '70s were hard to top; however, the '80s had their moments. Do you remember when ESPN started? It premiered in 1979 but the current logo, the one we all know and recognize, made its debut in 1985, and to me that was when it really started to become recognized. I spent a large chunk of the '80s tending bar, so this new network, with this crazy Australian rules football on at 11:00 at night, well it just could not last. I mean, Entertainment, Sports, Programing, Network... it could never work, or could it?

Television was on the back burner for me. I was becoming way too cool and way too busy working nights to watch sitcoms anymore. Well, maybe way too busy; I was never way too cool. There were still the blockbuster shows; there was this show—maybe you've heard of it—it was called "Cheers", and it was a huge hit. Funny how the top show of the '80s was based in a bar; looking back you could say a reflection of the times, for sure.

In 2002, Cheers was ranked No. 18 on TV Guide's 50 Greatest TV Shows of All Time. Cheers won 26 Emmy Awards (from 117 nominations). It was able to keep its top characters throughout its 11 seasons, survived the death of one cast member (Nicholas Colasanto as "Coach"), the swapping out of the female lead (Kirstie Alley for Shelley Long), and even spawned a hugely successful spinoff series with another co-star ("Frasier" with Kelsey Grammer). And as an unexpected side benefit, the site of the bar in Boston is now a tourist magnet.

Following closely behind, was another microcosm of the 80s, "Miami Vice" (1984-89), which *People* magazine stated "was the first show to look really new and different since color TV was invented." Unlike standard police procedures, the show drew heavily upon 1980s "New Wave" principles and music. The show became widely recognized for its heavy integration of music and visual effects to tell a story. With Don Johnson and Philip Michael Thomas, a couple of cool guy vice squad bad asses, some people could easily argue this show, "Miami Vice", deserves the top spot. It's hard to say, but it definitely had all of the '80s social issues: plenty of drugs, drinks, girls, fast cars and fast boats. It was a huge hit. Doing all of the bad things socially was glamorized; you were not cool unless you were snorting coke and swilling alcohol.

We had Tom Selleck as "Magnum PI", and "The Cosby Show", "The Dukes of Hazard" and "Night Court". Larry Hagman jumped from astronaut Major Anthony Nelson to J.R. Ewing in "Dallas", while Cybil Shepard and Bruce Willis formed a great team in "Moonlighting". How about a team like long-time star George Peppard sharing a show with Mr. T in the "A Team"? What a match! "Remington Steele" with Pierce Brosnan and Stephanie Zimbalist was big, and who could ever forget "Square Pegs", with youngster Sarah Jessica Parker. "The Love Boat", "Fantasy Island" and the classic "Pee Wee's Playhouse", (I mean how did this guy get a TV show anyway?) and don't forget "Soap"; that was television.

How about our music? This is something that continued to rival the '70s and because I was fully involved with the bar tending/bar manager gig I had to buy music for the clubs where I worked. Going to college, yes this is the first stint, and not to be the last; working nights made my knowing much about television programming kind of limited; however, I was right on the edge of the music scene. People I became friends with in So-Cal introduced me to this new genre called "New Wave", sort of a techno disco sort of style. There were of course the B-52s (I did see these guys at the Hollywood Bowl), and I didn't have a clue what "Rock Lobster" was. Hell, I called it "crab rock", and my buds thought that DEVO was big, as was Adam Ant, Blondie, and Big Country. Big Country's album "The Crossing", featuring the song (of all names) "In a Big Country", got played a ton in my DJ/bartending gig. Do you recall some of these? The Call, Duran Duran, Billy Idol, Peter Gabriel, and Joe Jackson swooned us with his songs of lost love, never found love and heartache. The Plimsouls were huge in my world, as was Oingo Boingo, the Tubes, the Romantics and Men at Work. Yes, Men at Work; they jammed in the club and got the girls up and dancing. I still listen to INXS, have their greatest hits on my iPod, and listen to a lot of these bands to this day. It's called longevity and creativity.

Michael Jackson's "Thriller" was released in 1982, and in just over a year it became—and currently remains—the best-selling album of all time, with sales projected by various sources at between 65 and 110 million copies globally, and is also tied for the best-selling album in the United States. This record won a record-breaking eight Grammy Awards at the 1984 Grammys, and the groove got wore of this bad boy on our portable DJ station at the club. The "Thriller" video was a trend-setting masterpiece; I must have played it hundreds of times on our three-gun projection big screen at the club. It was incredible.

Funk became mainstream and popular with bands like Herbie Hancock, Parliament, Kool and the Gang and the Gap Band. Funk was an extension of Motown, James Brown, Prince, and Wild Cherry. Stevie Wonder, Average White Band, The Commodores—of course featuring Lionel Ritchie, and "Brick House" was a classic. And what about Rose Royce and their tune "Car Wash", and "Low Rider" by War? With the color barrier broken down crossover tunes and genres were normalized; it didn't matter what color your skin was to me, if it thumped, bumped and could be played loud, then it was great.

And what about rap and its beginnings, the break into mainstream days? Run DMC, the Beastie Boys, and believe it or not Will Smith and his Fresh Prince were cool. LL Cool J, Grand Master Flash, Ice-T and the Sugar Hill Gang—all trendsetters and groundbreakers, building the foundation for the billion dollar rap industry of today.

There were Madonna, U2, Guns 'N Roses and Metallica, not to mention Van Halen, Tom Petty and Jackson Browne. Bruce Springsteen, remember him? The Cars, Journey, Boston , The Eagles and Bob Seger were still cranking out hits. ZZ Top, Foreigner, and Fleetwood Mac—some may have started in the '70s and carried through the '80s; I know there are many more and at some point I would love to compile a list of your favorites all together. MTV and music video were born, adding to the exposure of artists and music. Suffice to say the '80s were a great decade for music.

Motion pictures were becoming blockbusters with huge dramatics and special effects. "Close Encounters" and "E-T", "Star Wars" and "Star Trek", "Superman" and "Raiders of the Lost Ark" were big-budget, and even bigger money makers. I would gamble and say anyone reading this book saw every one of those films. Richard Pryor and Gene Wilder teamed up in "Stir Crazy", a follow-up from the '70s "Silver Streak". "Rocky III" featured Sly and Mr. T; in '85 Stallone had a good year with both "Rocky IV" and "Rambo", Mel Gibson and Danny Glover found gold with "Lethal Weapon", and "Ghost Busters" was massive. "Back to the Future", both One and Two were awesome. Who could not like Michael J. Fox? Along with "Ghostbusters" One and Two, sequels equated to big bucks and therefore follow-ups. "Raiders" had two, with "Indiana Jones" in '84 and a father-son sequel with Sean Connery in "Indiana Jones and the Last Crusade" in '89. Those three films alone grossed an estimated, mind-boggling, and staggering $580 million.

James Bond returned five times–yes, five—with Roger Moore (I always liked Roger, however Sean Connery is my fave) starring in "For Your Eyes Only" in '81, "Octopussy" in '83 (and by the way, what's with that title, anyway?) and "A View to a Kill" in '85. Timothy Dalton took over the speed boat and racecar for two films, starring in "The Living Daylights" in '87 and "License to Kill" in '89. Moore starred in a total of seven Bond films through the '70s and '80s, and my fave Connery only starred in 5, from the '60s and the '70s. I think it's the young boy memories that kind of sway my opinion; I would be curious to see a poll on boomer favorites – it would be interesting for sure.

Star Wars may have started in '79, however, the total number in the franchise is debatable. I found many results that claimed there were six total in the franchise and some opinions say there were eight; in any event it has become an industry upon itself, born of boomer money and boomer adulthood, so I lay claim to our demographic making it a success. So in essence George Lucas owes us, right?

Star Trek may have started their run the same year as Star Wars ('79) but they actually have them beat as far as a total number of productions with 11 films (as of 2009). There were four films in the 80s: "Star Trek II: The Wrath of Khan" (1982), "Star Trek III: The Search for Spock" (1984), "Star Trek IV: The Voyage Home" (1986), and "Star Trek V: The Final Frontier" (1989). In my opinion these were the preeminent films of this franchise; it really must be hard to continue to churn out quality, and frankly you have to give all of these franchises credit—they were good.

Batman reappeared in the '80s once, in a clever title: "Batman". There are a total of 11 Batman films spread throughout time starting in the 1940s; however, the reappearance of the Batmobile and Bruce Wayne occurred in '89.

"Superman", the first movie, premiered in 1978, with three installments in the 80s: "Superman II" in 1980,

"Superman III" in '83 and "Superman IV, The Quest for Peace" in '87, which finished the trifecta for the 80s. In all there were seven Superman films with the last installment, correctly titled "Superman Returns" arriving at theaters in 2006.

Bruce Willis' "Die Hard" films started in '89 and he played the role of John McClain four times. I guess it's like the old saying, "Ride the pony till the pony can't run anymore," with these franchises.

Obviously this is just a snapshot of the content generated in the '80s; in looking at the Top 10 lists while researching this section I was mildly surprised at how many of these films I had seen. I am sure I am not alone in the fact that we as boomers, which at this point in 1980 the oldest would have been 34 and the youngest would have been 16 (personally I was 21), that the gravitating away from the small screen to the big was normal. Especially considering that this could be considered the decade of the blockbuster, and the investment needed to recoup costs drove a marketing binge.

Social issues were always occurring, so it amazes me how we can view what is happening in today's culture and think that this is the so-called "be all, end all". History proves that once again we boomers lived through a turbulent time in the '80s. Between natural disasters, man-made disasters, political issues and human rights issues, evolution and experience are always on our side. We have lived through a lot, and learned how to endure.

I had not been in So-Cal very long (exact dates escape me), but I know I vividly remember Mt. Saint Helens blowing her stack and killing 57 people. Sometimes I wonder about all of that soot and gas that was pumped into the atmosphere, and I wonder if these kinds of occurrences contribute to our global warming... I digress, again, sorry. Mexico City had the 8.1 earthquake in

1985, which rocked Mexico, and the 1989 Loma Pietà, San Francisco quake caused billions in damage. Many remember this as the World Series quake; I do because I was coming home from work and was listening to the start of the game on the radio and I remember Al Michaels and his color analysis. On a side note, I would say that in my 15 years of living in So-Cal I experienced four or five big rockers (quakes), and frankly after the Northridge quake in '94 I had my fill and wanted out. In '95 I would return to Michigan as a single dad with a seven-year-old daughter. Earthquakes scare the crap out of me; they are unannounced visitors, and you just never know how long they are going to stay—seriously scary stuff.

In 1986 the Challenger disaster occurred, and again I saw this live, in an almost surreal moment. The Chernobyl meltdown occurred later that same year affecting hundreds of thousands. The worst single aviation loss of life occurred when Japan Airlines flight 123 crashed on August 12, 1985, killing all 520 people on board. The Soviets shot down a commercial airliner, Korean flight 007, on September 1, 1983, killing all 269 passengers. The Exxon Valdez ran aground in Alaska when the radar onboard failed to work (reportedly was broken), causing a major oil spill in the environmentally sensitive Prince William Sound. In 1984, the Bhopal catastrophe ensued from a toxic MIC gas leak at the Union Carbide plant in Bhopal, India, killing 3,000 immediately and ultimately claiming 15,000–20,000 lives.

Senseless deaths seemed to become common, if that is possible. John Lennon was shot and killed in 1980—an awful tragedy. In 1981 Egyptian President Anwar Sadat was killed, President Ronald Reagan was shot and injured by gunman John Hinckley, and Pope John Paul II had an attempt made on his life in Saint Peters Square. In 1984 we saw the death of the first female

Indian Prime minister, Indira Gandhi, gunned down by her own bodyguards. And singer Marvin Gaye was shot and killed by his own father, reportedly in a dispute over money. I personally took this loss with a heavy heart, being a huge fan of Gaye and his awesome music. All of these were senseless tragedies.

Technology was continuing to gain steam and court rulings would inevitably have a major impact on the world, but also touched me personally, bringing my telecom career to a beginning, although at that time I had no idea. The ruling by Judge Greene in 1982 to divest AT&T, which came to be known as the "breakup" in 1984, ushered in a whole new wave of technology and opened the door to the computer generation. It would be that same year, '84, that the first Macintosh computer was introduced. MS-Dos was introduced in the mid '80s; even though Microsoft may have been formed in the mid '70s it was actually in 1986 that 12,000 employees of the company became millionaires with their IPO. The mid '80s were explosive times as far as the advent of technology.

Arcade games, outgrowths of pinball, were growing in popularity in the late '70s; however, a glut of low-quality games caused the gaming market to crash in 1983. In the mid '80s this trend would rebound with the introduction of the Nintendo Entertainment System (NES), and they would eventually grab a reported 90% market share. I missed this whole wave of entertainment; I thought the arcade games were cool, but the television game systems and those handheld devices just never turned me on. To this day I find video games to be a complete waste of time; I am sure there are many younger people who would think this is heresy, even my younger brothers were into the gaming stuff, but I never got it and I now believe that this type of entertainment is actually one of the root causes of our childhood obesity issues.

Ronald Reagan was elected our President in 1980 and then was re-elected in 1984 in an overwhelming landslide. His policies, some credit with generating an ideological renaissance on the American political right, ushered in the fall of what he called the Soviet evil empire. His policy of abandoning détente and building up our military, which he coined the "Star Wars" defense system line, helped drive the Soviets to bankruptcy, which culminated with the fall of the Berlin wall in 1989 and ended the Cold War. It would be Reagan and his policies that would support anti-communist movements worldwide. His "Reaganomics", a supply-sided economic model, advocated controlling the money supply, reducing tax rates and the deregulation of the economy (recall the earlier "breakup" of AT&T), reducing government spending—all of which spurred economic growth. Reagan's presidency from 1980 until 1988 set the stage for growth and prosperity, and even though there were many social issues and aforementioned events, the '80s will be remembered as a golden era.

Is the behavior and abuse issue coming through loud and clear?

Meanwhile, back in school

Being a non-traditional student had its moments, and for a long time I avoided that term when referring to myself. But now as I reflect back on the whole process, I embrace the feeling of accomplishment, and let me remind you of something: Even though I took over twenty years off from school, when it was all said and done, here are the facts: It took me six years to finish an undergraduate degree (with honors by the way), three years to finish the Master's degree, and one year to prep and become certified as a personal trainer (frankly I had no prior anatomy or physiology training; I just liked working out). This adds up to 10 years. It was pretty ironic how, unbeknownst to me, this 10-year, 10,000-hour thing even existed, but once it became clear, it made writing this book and helping other boomers understand the quest, and why it is so important, become a passion, and I like to think destiny (sorry, Lo)!

15: Becoming Great

In discussing behavior, I believe that the key to anything we do starts and ends with motivation. Motivation holds the key; it is the drive to fulfill that desire and change, so it has been an area of interest to me for as long as I can remember. All of the good and bad behaviors I have lived through really all start with motivation first.

Being properly motivated is the difference between being outstanding, or simply average. You can be an average softball player, or you can be a Division One athlete in college—what's the difference? It's definitely motivation. Developing mastery in motivation requires a process, a game plan, a strategy. The more you invest in developing your skills, the higher the rewards will be. Remember the 10,000 hours or 10 years necessary to become an expert? Motivation is the overarching key to our success.

When I started writing my notes for this book I was motivated to share the whole story. When I quit the drinking and the drug use, it was motivation. When I made the decision to jump back into school and finish that first degree, it was motivation. Motivation led the getting in shape, the changing of the diet, the bodybuilding show, the starting of a side business, the forming of our mastermind group, the radio talk show, really everything. You see—more and more items, they started to stack up, the goals started to be accomplished, the re-thinking and moving forward with new mountains to climb, all due to motivation.

So motivation is the overarching behavior; it is the strategic point of it all. Let's start with four main topics and build from there:

- Motivation is intrinsic; it must start from within the individual.

- Understand the difference in positive and negative motivation and that everyone already is motivated in some way, just maybe not in the best way to find success.

- People will do things for their own self-interest. I can't tell you that you need to work out or lose weight, but I can share the benefits of the compelling "WHY" you should, and help you learn, if you want to.

- Understand the needs of the person whom we want to help, and build on those; everyone is essentially different.

Changing perspective

As we move through our lives there are those many ups and downs that we all experience, some troubling, some not so; however, it is how we adjust our behavior that makes all the difference in our future. Obviously we cannot change the past, but we can learn, and hopefully we do. I know I did, which is why I want to share this short intro before we put our heads down and plow into the next section.

Sandy

Having gone through a divorce and being a single dad for many years, my whole thought process on relationships was totally hosed. A product of a broken family myself as a youth, going through a marriage failure seemed at the time much more than I wanted to deal with; the thought of despair and 'loser-ness' was like a boulder on my back. Looking back it was a perfect excuse for some of the destructive behavior that I exhibited; "Oh, woe is me" should have been my anthem; what a dumbass. Luckily for this dumbass loser something or someone (I can get into divine intervention, but just bear with me for a minute), helped get my proverbial head out of my ass and quit being a self-centered downer.

I understand everyone has these ups and downs in life; it's called growing up. It just takes some of us longer. Anyway, the point is—without going into a long drawn-out journey of self-pity and 'crybaby-ness' (these new words, I hope the message is clear)—it really was about behavior change, and that is the point of this intro. Having gone through that marriage failure (truly a blessing in disguise), I had the chance to wallow, raise my daughter, and wallow some more. By that I mean I was anti-relationship, anti-establishment, anti-marriage and/or dating, no way, no how. And this went on for several years... actually more like six or seven, now that I actually think about it.

I had somehow discovered that a girl I had dated in high school (whom I had always had kind of a high-school memory crush on), was single and not married. I had heard that she had married, had a child and so on, you know the routine. Anyway, much to my delight, I learned she had not married, did have a child, but was single, as was I. It took some time to 'grow a pair' and make the reach-out call, (remember that this was almost 25 years since I had dated this girl in high school, and we had had zero contact), but I did. She barely remembered me, was very nice, was leaving on vacation and would call me when she returned, great, awesome, fantastic, except the call never came. That figures; chalk it up to another strikeout.

Hold on, remember someone, or something, had bigger plans for me. Three months went by and then—voila, she called. I have to give her mother credit for planting that seed. It seems that she was dating someone when I originally called, and was too nice to blow me off, so she gave me the nice girl, "I will call you when I get home" line, and now 'boyfriend' was history, so mother convinced daughter to call me back. There are more details to this, but suffice to say that we arranged our initial date for the following weekend. Talk about apprehension... 25 years can produce a number of changes—ever been to a 20-year class reunion? You catch my drift.

When date night came, she actually picked me up (she had a nicer vehicle and maybe she wanted her escape vehicle ready); let me tell you—and this is the honest truth, when this woman got out of her van, I was stunned! She looked the same as she did in high school, a total knockout doll! I was more than stunned. I was knocked for a loop.

It was the beginning of my new life. Eight months later, we were married, and it was a complete blessing. She is my guide, my stabilizer, my friend and my lover.

Ok, so I made this short, but long enough to get the message I hope, and that is never lose that mental attitude of being positive for change; be open and willing, because behavior is everything and things can be modified if you want them to; I did, and so can you.

Section 2:

Behavior

This section of the book is, by far, the most important of the entire text; how we think, how our brain processes work, and how we react are completely up to us.

16: List things out

A positive attitude, access to correct infor-mation, and a like-minded circle of friends is more important than any amount of will power for accomplishing goals and improving your life.

In the perpetual Indian summer of our lives, we need to find ourselves. We de-serve to feel alive and look forward to our futures. We boomers have a LOT of life to live. This is a special time that has been earned through all of the efforts of grow-ing up—yes, growing up. We never stop this process. Growing up is a continual development. There is no magic number. What we have done is invested in our lives and those around us, and we have paid for this investment with our first careers, children, experiences and we now move to the next phase; isn't it great to think in this way, continually working toward the improvement of our QOL?

Mindset is the key, and behavior is the engine that drives mindset. This section is devoted to suggestions for those behaviors; I wish it could be all-inclusive, but it is not. However, it is a compilation of behaviors that have helped this ordinary guy accomplish some extraordinary goals, and with picking and choosing the suggestions I have listed, you surely can make a difference in your life journey. I look forward to building on this list and with your suggestions sharing behaviors with many others in the future.

That's the beauty of the radio talk show "Boomers Rock". It gives all of us a forum to share ideas by either listening and learning, or writing or calling in.

It is that collective mindset of helping others that will move us forward; that is what 200% is all about. It is why boomers truly do rock!

Pulling the trigger

Much more has been written about the anatomy and physiology of our magnificent brains; my purpose is to blend all of it together and try and instill that desire to improve, to basically share what this ordinary boomer has done. I have learned and accomplished and want to instill in you the belief that anything is possible. Now that we have learned the three key components of our brain, neurogenesis, neuroplasticity, and myelin, it is time to move into the really fun stuff: behavior.

Many Baby Boomers will face wellbeing issues. Many will simply not have the wherewithal—financial, emotional, logistical—to make critical changes in their lives. We will be required to face up to these and many other difficult encounters, life is a journey for sure.

The Top Ten

My buddy from California, Dr. Ray Faulkenberry, is someone who, once you talk to him, you'll consider one of your best friends. Ray told me to come up with my list. It sounds like an easy assignment but you must become focused—you have to define things.

1. Imagination—"Whatever the mind can conceive and believe we can achieve." Inside imaginations are dreams, and through the whole process we need to visualize everything. You have to be able to see it, before you can achieve it.

2. Goals—especially Big, Hairy, Audacious, Goals. With goals you have the definitiveness of purpose, establishing short-, medium- and long-term goals, with laser-like FOCUS. With goals you have to think big; again, see it, verbalize your goals, write them down, and strategize. There is no playing around with goals; you have to map them, practice them, plan for them, and attack them. Think of goals as our overarching mission statement; did I mention I love goals? More on this later.

3. Faith/Belief—confidence, success, sense of purpose, believe and achieve, limiting negative beliefs and giving of yourself; the sense of something bigger than you pushing your sail, spirituality

4. Positive Mental Attitude (PMA), Entanglement and quantum physics, PEN (Positive Energy Network), perspective, strength, practice. NET (Negative Energy Tornado), dream-killer, second guessing, hopelessness

5. Happiness—Eternally optimistic, the meaning of life, sharing and giving, health and vitality, (practice)

6. Habits—Our "Path in the Grass," as Dr. Lori Shemeck says, brain mapping, good versus bad and understanding why, sledding down a hill (Passionate Practice)

7. Fear—Of success and of failure/stressors

8. Love—Yourself and then others, how, why, when, who, self-esteem

9. Enthusiasm—Being "all-in", motivation

10. Catalyst—The trigger

17: Imagination

It all starts with imagination, that ability to throw your mind so wide open that anything is possible. Albert Einstein was quoted as saying, "Imagination is more important than knowledge. For knowledge is limited to all we know and understand, while imagination embraces the entire world and all we know and understand." Napoleon Hill followed that with his description of imagination as, "the most miraculous incomprehensible force that the world has ever known." It is like the brain-mapping, myelin-building, and neuroplasticity-changing phenomenon, "use it or lose it rule"; to build it and get better, think about something extraordinary, or "day dream", as Dr. Oz said.

Imagination stretches our minds and it is the pinnacle of thought; like Einstein wrote, "imagination is more important than knowledge."

So let's step back for just a second and talk about one more component of our brain, the reticular activating system, or RAS.

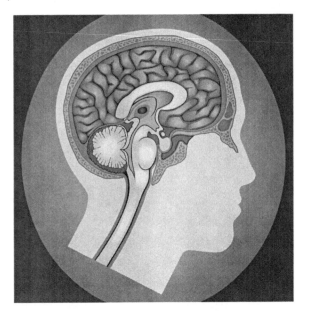

The Reticular Activating System, or RAS[vii], coordinates all brain and body activities to maintain homeostasis (think of our built-in ability to maintain a stable state) in all our physiological, biological, bio-sociological, psychological, emotional, and volitional states.

The RAS generates all autonomic responses, including all emotions, response-impulses, and in the healthy brain, all psychopathologies. In other words, the RAS is our filter to our world, our conscious and unconscious information filtering, some 100 million impulses per second—and we are aware of perhaps one percent of those impulses. I like to think of the RAS as the great refrigerator door of our brain; if you are not programmed to accept the information, your RAS automatically filters it out and those unconscious and conscious thoughts never make it to first base, or the light in the refrigerator never comes on.

This is the most awesome thing about the RAS and why it is important, even critical to our improvement and success. If we can create a clear picture in our mind, we are opening the refrigerator door. If we cannot imagine it, if our RAS does not feel there is a need for our brain to accept the impulse, the bits of information, the string of information is filtered out and we are never aware of the stimulus; it happens every day, all the time. If we did not have this refrigerator door protecting our three-pound muscle, our brain, we would blow the motherboard and, like a hard drive failure, shut down the operating system... not good.

If you can imagine it, you can achieve it; you are not restricted in any way, and there are no rules, only your own "Refrigerator Door"!

Imagination is much more important than many people realize. Creative imagination is one of the most powerful tools we own, and it is ours to use as we see fit. Imagination creates the picture, and if our RAS has been told to allow the picture into our subconscious, it can take place. We behave in ways that our brain has been conditioned for; it allows us to act or fail to act dependent upon our imagination.

It is not will, but imagination.

Why is it that when people are hypnotized to believe they are cold, for example, their temperature drops? It is because our nervous system cannot tell the difference between imagined experience and real experience; it is the RAS working automatically. Automatic behaviors and subconscious reactions are constantly occurring. Our brain is built in such a way (remember the RAS is our filter) to react automatically to stress; it is the saber-toothed tiger, caveman DNA—we react, adjust, and function, all to protect ourselves.

Emotional reactions to stimuli are the intrinsic unconscious reaction to learned stimuli; it is the thought, real or simply perceived, that triggers the response. The same thing occurs with a negative thought; exactly the same thing can occur if our filter (RAS) allows it to pass into our subconscious.

Imagination is the canvas of our mind, where we can paint the picture, in any color, any shade. It is where we can combine old ways of doing things with the well-established infrastructure and continue to expand, like a telephone network and its central office, the hub. You will never have that major purpose in your life, you will never achieve confidence in your abilities, become a leader of men and women, unless you can first create these qualities in your mind—and your imagination is the key.

Dreams are fed from your imagination; ideas are born from your imagination; goals are started within your imagination, and it all starts with your canvas and how you want the picture to look. Steve Jobs and Steve Wozniak saw in their imaginations a user-friendly, small, sleek tool called a personal computer, and although all of the high-rollers of the computer industry scoffed at these upstarts they persisted, forged ahead with the idea, and set their goal to build it, and Apple computer was conceived.

You own your imagination; it is in your soul—stand up and see it. Nothing was ever created by a human being that was not first the product of someone's imagination. If you continue to paint the picture, your canvas will develop the picture and soon, through constant effort and persistence, achievement will occur.

I never had any idea that I would go to graduate school; my refrigerator door, my RAS, was completely closed to the possibility. I was still mad at myself for not finishing college with people my own age, way back in the '80s. But a strange thing started to occur: I kept working at it, and you know what? I got better; it started to come together for me and my imagination started to kick into gear; things started changing. Instead of being the introverted, self-deprecating old guy I started to grow confidence, and with that came excitement and momentum. Students started to want to be in my group; I started leading, and school was becoming less of a downer and much more of an uplifting effort. I wanted to improve; I wanted to encourage.

Inspire people with a vision that is exciting to follow. One trait common to all leaders is VISION, and vision can only come from imagination! My RAS had started to change, and my refrigerator door was open; the light was on to so many options—it truly was amazing.

Newsweek magazine reported in August of 2010, in an article titled, "The Golden Age of Innovation," that the largest group of entrepreneurship has shifted to the 55- to 64-year-old age group. Why? Individuals over 55 are reportedly nearly twice as likely to build successful companies as our counterparts in the millennial demographic (20- to 30-year-olds).

It is imagination that will fuel growth. That, and Boomer experience.

What if:

- you found a business model, health plan, exercise routine and mindset that could help others, building their self-worth and increasing their quality of life?

- you were in a position to be a pioneer in a network of people who are changing the way we live, teach and help our younger generations?

- you could develop future leaders to help push "The Flywheel", by encouraging skill development, outreach and care, which could change people's lives?

- you became part of a grassroots effort that makes examples of ordinary people?

- you set the pace, explain, teach and then demonstrate how to do it?

- you went back to your beliefs with the opportunity, realistic expectations, and genuine desire to teach and help your prospects – could you build a stable organization?

And what if:

- people judged you by your appearance, which of course they do, and you projected a positive image, confidence, and were self-assured?

- you are excited about what you do—will you expect others to be excited also?

- you want it, believe in it, know you deserve it, and do what you must to achieve it?

It's called "Boomers Rock" for a reason!

Imagination + Visualization + Positive Thoughts all multiplied by Action = Success

Virtually all great accomplishments began in someone's imagination. For maximum achievement, you must mix effort with imagination. This is an area where your mastermind group is especially helpful.

18: Goals

We have already talked about my love for goals – but let's delve a bit deeper into WHY I love goals, the importance of goals.

A research study was conducted at Harvard University to determine what happens to students who set goals. A survey was conducted with 100 students, and it was discovered that only five of those 100 set goals on a regular basis, in a logical manner. Upon a follow-up study with the same 100 students, it was determined that the five percent who had established their logical goals had achieved 93 percent of the net worth of the entire group; the remaining 95 only had seven percent of the net worth.

Understand that financial net worth is not the only measure of success. The survey went deeper and discovered that the original five (goal setters) were more satisfied with their family life, were in better physical condition, were in higher positions of authority in their jobs, and emotionally were more at peace with themselves and their families.

Goal setters are winners!

BHAGs

The term Big Hairy Audacious Goal ("BHAG") was proposed by James Collins and Jerry Porras in their 1996 article entitled "Building Your Company's Vision." A BHAG encourages companies to define visionary goals that are more strategic and emotionally compelling.

In the article, the authors define a BHAG (pronounced BEE-hag) as a form of vision statement "...an audacious 10- to 30-year goal to progress towards an envisioned future."

A true BHAG is clear and compelling, serves as unifying focal point of effort, and acts as a clear catalyst for team spirit. It has a clear finish line, so the organization can know when it has achieved the goal; people like to shoot for finish lines.[15]

Why is it that so many people have that desire for change? Really, they want to, but nothing ever happens? It's the way we approach goals; we have been conditioned. As an infant we have only that desire for fulfillment; there were no inhibitions, we were a blank slate who cried when we wanted something. It was not until we grew older that the experience of "No" started to occur:

- That's not good for you!

- Don't do that!

- Don't be such a baby—stop crying!

- Don't touch that!

- I said, "No"!

Coaching kids is great training for coaching adults, because they can more easily see the short term, they haven't been soured on the upward mobility of life, and they just want to be coached and experience fun. Why are adults getting ready to start all the time but never pull the trigger? Let me tell you: it's bad goal setting, or for that matter, *no* goal setting. Do not fret, because we are in the perfect place to capitalize on our wisdom and knowledge and frankly, the world needs us boomers.

I like this way of describing goals, this is how we start:

- Writing and sharing—Verbalize your goals; share with your family, your friends and your co-workers. Make them real to your RAS, write them down, start the brain mapping and let the neurogenesis begin; start building the myelin. The only way to start is to tell someone and then write it down for yourself; think about short, medium and long term. I have dry-erase boards everywhere: in the lab (err, basement gym), in the kitchen, in the computer room, three or four in the studio, everywhere. It makes it really easy to put that thought down, that piece of inspired genesis of an idea, because they are fleeting. And if they are clearly on display around the house, anyone who comes into that room can see what you are doing; it's no secret.

- See it, own it, visualize it—again, this is another key brain technique. Understand where imagination comes into play? You must see yourself doing it, working toward it, planning for it and getting it done. Close your eyes and picture every goal, believe you have attained it, get that feeling deep down, and start thinking about that follow-up goal, the "if so, now what?" feeling.

- Become energized—Lose the doubt, focus on the BHAG, but let's do it in a logical way, so as to give yourself that fighting chance. I carry a card in my wallet, one of those ideas that success-ful people do; it is right there whenever I open the wallet—my biggest, most important of all BHAGs. I smile when I see the card–heck, I can't even remember when I wrote it, but it doesn't matter; it's there.

The journey of going back to college was a long pro-cess, but you have to have the three steps, and the short-, medium- and long-term map ready. Many "over-night" success stories really were not overnight. Many spent years toiling, building their businesses or work-ing toward the end result. Preparation takes time. You don't become an All-American or an All-Pro overnight.

Going back to school —Unfinished business

It can't be emphasized enough how important the life-long education process has become to me, and should be for you. It really is quite clear now that there are many factors that can help people of all ages, but more impor-tantly for us boomers. That cognitive decline and men-tal illness could potentially be held off, if not avoided all together, by continuing to learn. It is critical.

I can say personally that I feel extremely blessed to have had the good fortune to go back to college at 40 years old and spend the next nine years sweating it out with the traditional students. That, unbeknownst to me at the time and completely accidental, I was helping my cognitive skills by taking all of those classes. That at this point in my life, with the improvements in diet and exercise, my capacity to learn and take on new challenges was a not-so-coincidental byproduct of college as an old guy. Who could have known that the original process of all of the "coincidental" actions that were occurring were, in fact, because the idea for becoming an entrepreneur and/or messenger was, in fact, the seed planted during college. That is one key reason I encourage anyone to consider going back and taking a class or two. Give it a try; you never know what may happen. I will always be a supporter of anyone who wants to give it a shot, and coach you up if you want—no problem!

One of the problems the Baby Boomers have bequeathed to the millennial and Gen Y generations is their reliance on quick fixes, instantaneous gratification and their dependence on technology. This is another area where boomers can excel in the perpetual "Indian summers" of their lives: sharing and teaching younger people how to be patient. They do not realize that having a target in their life can have a tremendously synergistic effect on their existence, and achievement of long-term goals. Training and learning all of this education has a tremendous impact on our goals, and our achievement. It is imperative.

See the value in building the foundation, the short-term goals, the six- to twelve-month goal—this is a short-term goal. You would not build a house without a solid foundation, would you? It is the first step up the mountain; all of the fundamentals we need to be successful are achieved in our short-term plan. You are setting the stage for your victory; remember, we have the best work ethic of any generation.

Next are the medium goals, the toughest of the three. Medium goals take the fortitude; however, if you understand and plan for the long-term you will realize that the medium goals can be kind of fun, because we begin to arrive at our cruise-control speed; we are past the foundation, we know that we are putting up the framing of our house and things are starting to take shape. If you could not see the end result before, you should start to very soon.

Science experts, neuropsychologists, and other experts on success know the brain is a goal-seeking organism. Whatever your subconscious mind has developed in your goal-pursuing agenda, it will work day and night to achieve and fulfill.

Long-term goals, the big picture, that college degree, the new training has been completed and that new job is right around the corner, the next chapter is ready to begin. That's the total beauty of the three sets of goals—big things, big doors, windows of opportunity; everything starts to crystalize, all because you had that laser-like focus on the goals, and success comes to those who persevere.

Use these steps:

1. Goals should be clearly stated: You have to be able to define and articulate what it is you want to accomplish. If I say my goal is to travel more, this is too vague and will not stimulate me to go further. It is more powerful if I state that my goal is to spend six months traveling the United States by motorhome. Now, I can begin to formulate a plan on how much money this will require, and the details I need to look into to make it happen. Be specific!

2. Goals should be inspiring: If your goal is something that is completely new to you, you need it to inspire you. Without inspiration you will not have the energy to take action. Your goal should cause you to have feelings of excitement, joy, and enthusiasm.

3. Goals should be measurable: Develop a clear picture, visualize what you want, think about the possible ways you can make it happen, take action, and then measure the results. Keep working at it, take action, learn along the way, fine tune and adjust your actions for maximum return on your energy and investment.

4. Goals should be action-based: When you take action, you are fully present in whatever you are doing, and you keep working, climbing the mountain. Complete actions will yield the necessary results to your desired outcome. Comprehensive and total actions are mental, physical, emotional, and spiritual in nature.

5. Goals should be written down: It's not real until you write it down. Be very specific and put your goals where you will be able to reference them regularly. I carry a note card in my wallet; many successful people do the same, so start!

6. Goals should be shared with as many people as possible; don't be afraid of criticism or doubters— count on it and shrug it off. Make yourself accountable; you are more likely to take action if you put yourself out there and let people know about your goals.

7. Goals should be flexible: Life is not linear; it's dynamic. Things are going to change. You will find out many things on your journey, so you must have the flexibility to change. You might find out that the things you thought you wanted did not really serve your higher purpose, or they might lead to something completely new.

> Your subconscious mind does not argue with you. It accepts what your conscious mind decrees. If you say "I can't afford it," your subconscious mind works to make it true. Select a better thought. Decree, "I'll buy it. Accept it in my mind.
>
> ~Dr. Joseph Murphy

19: Faith

The band Fleetwood Mac (perfect for us boomers) bounce around like so many bands of the '70s, reinventing themselves, experimenting, mixing, changing it up, anything from reggae, party music, blues, and then they find the right combo. Their 15th album sold more than 4 million copies, and their 16th broke the bank. "Rumors" (great album) sold more than 19 million copies—which at that point in history was the number one-selling album in history. As Malcolm Gladwell wrote, (*"Outliers", Malcolm Gladwell, Little Brown and Company 2008)* "The band's original members are literally onto their third marriage. They have kids in high school. Their hair is gray. They have IRAs." It really came down to faith, because without it there is no way.

In my original notes this chapter was going to be called, "It's the hand of God that is guiding my life." I was very nervous about writing this, really. I think deep down I was afraid of my own feelings.

Sharing is hard sometimes, but it can be therapeutic, and I wanted to be as completely honest as possible. Being raised in the Catholic religion, and Catholic school for a good portion of my elementary years, those values were all I knew. I had never walked into or attended another service until I was an adult, so that is all I had experienced. My faith in a higher being has never wavered, even though I am not a go-to-church kind of person—I want to emphasize that. As life continued to unfold, goals continued to be met, accomplishments, and change, I started to wonder about the possibility of a higher being helping guide the way. All of the fantastic things that had been occurring the last oh, lifetime, or so, something had to be protecting me, guiding me. I mean frankly, when the 50th birthday hit I was completely thrilled just to be alive! It couldn't be luck, which is something that I don't believe in; luck is good planning, goals, achievement, and last but not least, faith.

Believing in yourself is completely attitude.

If I wanted to be successful in creating that next chapter in my life it was going to be through faith in what I was doing, understanding this, and that we can make a difference. Believing in ourselves is of paramount importance; we are capable of making it happen, any dream, vision, BHAG, but we need to be focused. Whether you call it self-assurance, self-esteem, or self-confidence, it all comes down to that deep, inherent, intrinsic feeling of belief, the faith that it can be done, that we can do it. It takes this plus your belief in your own talent, life skills and wisdom.

In his autobiography "Pizza Tiger"[16] (as quoted by Clement in "Believe and Achieve"[17]), Tom Monaghan discussed his success and his relationship with his faith. "I know I can never be a success on this Earth unless I am on good terms with God," the former CEO and founder of Domino's Pizza stated. "My background makes concern about spiritual matters as natural to me as breathing. I grew up in a Catholic orphanage, and for a short time attended a seminary, with every intention of becoming a priest." Mr. Monaghan attributes much of his success to his strong spiritual beliefs and faith. "I know I would not have been able to build Domino's without the strength I gained from my religious faith. In the earlier years, I hit a series of difficulties. Each one seemed like a knockout blow. But I was able to get off the floor every time and come back stronger than ever. That's the power of faith. I use it every day. No matter how tense or tired I get, I can take time out to pray or say a rosary and feel refreshed. That's a tremendous asset."

Faith is one of the most important of human characteristics, without which we would be hard-pressed to accomplish anything. Without faith, accomplishing our goals would be very difficult. Faith is the glue that holds all religious beliefs together; without faith they all would crumble. No one can prove the existence of any higher being; for that matter no one can see electricity—we can't see it or touch it, but through our faith we can believe and count on accomplishments and turning on the lights. Business could not take place without faith in our sense that we will receive what we are seeking in a transaction. Buying a product online would not occur unless we had faith in the system. Faith, belief and confidence, the building on your sense of purpose, is the nature of our beings. As a boomer I continue to grow and apply what I have been blessed to learn, because something much larger than me is guiding this ship. It is the acceptance of this belief that continues to energize my desire to build, write and give. What else is there? Believe in yourself, and watch what happens.

20: Limiting Beliefs

Limiting beliefs are negative thoughts that can sabotage our efforts; there are no stress-free solutions. The best way to conquer limiting beliefs is through experience and defeat—yes, defeat. That is another of the qualities that makes boomers so powerful: the understanding and wisdom of time; we cannot waste it or disregard our talent and history. Every problem we have solved, every obstacle we have overcome, gives us the confidence and skill to achieve our goals. We have all made mistakes, still do, and probably always will—so what? Defeat is temporary, just a pebble on the road.

Do any of these negative beliefs ring a bell to you?

- You can't make that kind of money.

- Women just don't do that type of work.

- I can't apply for that job; they would never hire me.

- I won't ever accomplish anything in my life.

- Nothing I do is right.

You can overcome ANY limiting belief. You are capable and your time is worth the effort. Try this exercise the next time a limiting belief starts messing with you, your faith or your abilities:

- Limiting thought—I am not worthy of focusing on my own needs.

- Rebuttal—My needs are just as important, and I am worthy of improvement.

- Limiting thought—If I share my true feelings about this, people will think I am weak.

- Rebuttal—The more I express my true feelings, the more respect people will have of me.

- Limiting thought—There is no way I can go back to school and learn; it has been too long.

- Rebuttal—It is never too late, and educators love having students who are actually trying to learn.

- Limiting thought—I will never be able to lose that weight.

- Rebuttal—If I stick to my plan, small steps every day, I will accomplish my goal.

The inner you, your subconscious, needs affirmation. Build yourself up with where and what you want to accomplish. Turn a limiting belief into a catalyst for change, empower yourself and move toward your goals. Here is another exercise to help turn the limiting belief into a positive:

1. My limiting belief is_____

2. How does this belief disable my goal?

    _____

3. I want to feel, be, or act like

    _____

4. I give myself permission to change and feel good about myself by doing_____

Achievement is always more fulfilling when your mind believes in what you are doing. Faith is another word for belief, so faith is something we condition our minds to accept and appreciate. The term "autosuggestion" has been in existence for a long time; autosuggestion is a psychological technique that was developed by apothecary Émile Coué from the late 19th century to the early 20th century and is a very powerful tool to enhance your beliefs. Your belief is the element that determines the accomplishment of your subconscious mind. A mind dominated by positive thoughts and emotions becomes a favorable home for improvement; it is the leader of change.

As I came to understand my faith, the belief in what was occurring in sharing my story, I remembered Jim Collins's book *Good to Great ("Good to Great", Jim Collins, Harper Collins, 2001),* in which he spoke of pushing the flywheel. Personally, I like to think of pushing the boulder. Pushing the boulder is my analogy of the big goal, the dream, the vision and the imagination. As you lean on the boulder nothing happens; my faith in moving this huge object is non-existent. But I keep pushing, because I believe that this is the right thing to do, and I want this to happen, really badly. You just keep reinforcing your behavior, doing the right things, thinking the right thoughts, keeping the positive attitude, never giving up on the belief and the stone starts to move, ever so slowly. Keep using the autosuggestion, because faith is the only antidote to failure; faith is power, so the stone continues to move. Whatever my mind can conceive, I can achieve, and I am going to keep pushing, keep believing, keep putting out the extraordinary effort necessary to fulfill my dream, so my sense of purpose grows, and the stone gains momentum.

Now things start to get interesting; as I think back on many effects in the past I start to realize and believe that all of this was a master plan, that the higher order was in fact guiding my ship. Quitting the destructive behaviors, going back to college, becoming reacquainted with Sandy and getting married, starting graduate school, becoming ill, starting our fitness business, the body building show, the radio show, and now writing this book—all of this is the stone moving, the faith in sharing the message that ordinary people can change and improve. You can do those extraordinary things if you just believe; this is powerful stuff and it is the right time for all of us. Boomers need to think about all of this and dig deep and give back, because we are at a major crossroads in our history.

A classic definition of faith from Dr. Joseph Murphy from his classic *The Power of your Subconscious Mind*[18] is written as this:

> "Faith is, in a sense, accepting as true what
> your reason and senses deny, i.e., a shutting out
> of the little, rational, analytical, conscious mind

and embracing an attitude of complete reliance on the inner power of your subconscious mind. Faith as mentioned in the Bible is a way of thinking, an attitude of the mind, an inner certitude, knowing that the idea you fully accept in your conscious mind will be embodied in your subconscious mind and made manifest."

Let me close the faith section with this thought: When the farmer plants the seed, does he have faith in the growth of that plant? Think about that.

21: The 90's and beyond:

The beginning of the nineties was a continuation of the lost decade of the 80's. As I now understand old habits, yes they are slow to break. The alcohol abuse continued to escalate, the "recreational" drug use was more than recreational, my marriage finally did implode and by the middle of the decade I was ready to escape the "beautifulness" of So-Cal. Frankly it had become not so beautiful.

I need to digress for a moment, (surprise). This term "recreational" drug use is such a farce. I think that some master branding agent from Columbia must have coined that one, it gave all of us a justification for destructive behavior. I am not trying to avoid accountability, hardly, however there really is no such thing as "recreational". Metaphorically it is like saying you did not inhale, bullshit. Excusing behavior that you know is wrong is simply stupid and it is wrong, own it. It is one of my parachutes of excuses, and as you have read I had them all, in case I was pushed from the plane. Acknowledging the problem is the first step in recovery, that's all.

Oh and the money you waste on these destructive behaviors, yes it all adds up. Maybe you are like me and escape the long arm of the law, (which luckily I never had any issues with), and do not have to pay all of the extras for your sins. Count your blessings, because there are plenty of people who ruined their lives, careers, marriages, families, all for the love of the buzz. Recovery is sweet, and it is doable.

By 1995 I had spent a solid 15 years in So-Cal, it was time to run for the border. Not only was I approaching my 35th birthday, but having experienced several earthquakes, (the Northridge quake hit January 17th, 1995) I was so done with So-Cal. Or maybe So-Cal was so done with my sorry ass, as the youngsters say, "whatever". Ashley and I, (I was now a full custody single dad to a seven year old) filled a 72 Ford van up with as much of our stuff as we could cram into it and made a week-long trip back to the Midwest, it was February of 1995.

I was so clueless that I had actually kind of forgotten that it was probably pretty cold in the heartland in February. Poor little Ashley did not have any boots, a winter coat, gloves anything. It must have been quite the site when this 35 year old hippie looking long hair walked into a Wal-Mart somewhere in Missouri to buy winter gear. The clerks looked at me like I was some kind of freak, and guess what, they don't sell much winter clothing by that time of the year, they are gearing up for Easter and Spring, so we had to really dig to get this kid some semblance of warm clothes, have I said I was a dumbass enough? Anyway—

We made it back to Lansing, and began the new life that would evolve into where we are today. I thank my family, especially my brother Jim and his wife Amy for letting us live with them for three months while we figured things out. It took some time to readjust, and the alcohol abuse would continue until 1998, but things were slowly starting to come around. It takes time; when we talk about small steps I really mean it. But finally we landed, and the vicious spiral, my own negative energy tornado, was slowing down.

Many of the full on stories throughout the book now encapsulate post moving back to Michigan, single-dadness, becoming a former rather than a current user, going back to school, finding and reconnecting with Sandy, etc. It has been a process, and in retrospect made me what I am today, and in the progression of writing this first book I have embraced the sharing of this story, life is full of roller-coaster like dips and turns. But the funny thing is the train comes back to the station, you get off and start making decisions all over again, it never ends.

Every day is a new chapter to embrace, every day holds new potential. As you start to string everything together you have a journey. Yes like Lewis and Clarke wondering through the wilderness it can be a struggle, but the beauty of it all is change is doable, and quality of life is achievable, just never give up on the quest, believe!

> The only things that stand between a person and what they want in life are the will to try it and the faith to believe it's possible.
>
> ~Rich DeVos

22: My Demon— Alcohol

I want to share another part of my life with you; it was my belief that I could get better that helped me to make this change. Here it is:

My epiphany with my illness, the lightning strike of April 2008, was actually preceded with an earlier, somewhat similar experience. Yes, lightning can strike twice! It takes a trip down memory lane, stepping into the time machine for this one. For a minute let's revisit 1998.

It was in that year that I made the decision to quit drinking alcohol. I knew in my heart of hearts that I was drinking too much; however, I did not understand the complexities of alcoholism and problem drinking. But I knew I was not right.

I used on a daily basis, and frankly looked forward to getting done with work to get home and "relax". Sounds kind of funny to write this now some 13 years later; I believe that writing and sharing has always been in someone's grand plan. Not mine—I am just the messenger, but someone much larger than myself. Anyway...

When I wrote a two-part blog on what I titled "My Demon Alcohol" I had no idea that anyone would read it; it became, in our fledgling blogosphere, a big hitter. Dang, obviously this message needs to be shared.

Back to 1998, July 27th to be exact. I made the call, the decision to quit, and I did. Done, fini, close the door. No problem. However, now I had this nagging question: Shoot, if I can just quit like this—is there a problem?

Well, of course there was and I knew it, but it was going to take a lot more unraveling to understand the complexities. At that point I had never heard of "problem drinking", only the dreaded alcoholism. I attended AA meetings, and did the "admitting" to the group; however, I could tell there was a difference between what I was going through and what the people in the meetings were experiencing. I knew I was not being honest when I said, "Hi, I'm Tom, and I'm an alcoholic." Confusion and once again the hiding—I did not like the feeling. I thought it would be liberating to attend a meeting and meet with others in my situation; however, I hated the feeling of not fitting in. What the hell was wrong with me? These poor people are addicted, so what the heck was my deal? I needed help from someone.

I have no idea what made me think about calling my personal physician and asking for a referral to a counselor; I had never seen a counselor, but I knew deep down that I had some major issues. Again, that feeling of someone else's grand plan. I knew I was messed up, but just could not figure it out, not on my own.

I entered counseling, and let me say this right now—it was the BEST THING that I could have ever done.

I needed the faith to get better, because I surely had the desire. I was sick and tired of where I had evolved, and deep down I knew I needed help. No one enters counseling without apprehension; I mean, it's counseling, right? Nervous? Well, yeah. Here I am 38 years old, a single dad with a then 11-year-old daughter, with an admitted drinking issue, a recreational drug user. I mean, they take kids away from people with mental issues, right? Lock you up, padded room, right?

Um, not hardly, Cowboy.

My counselor, Dr. Pat Long, is a great guy. So here is another of the many funny things that can happen in someone's life, and I do not mean funny ha-ha, funny like odd. Dr. Long, on the referral from my personal doctor and great friend Tom Jamieson, was a forensic psychologist; he did not really see individual patients. He was a specialist, but for some reason, maybe as a favor to Dr. J. or maybe because he had pity on my sorry ass, he took me on as a patient. Oh, and did I mention I did not have insurance for this kind of care? Nope, out of pocket. And Dr. Long still took me on, God bless him.

What occurred in the next six to eight months (gosh it's been a long time so I don't actually recall exactly how long I saw Pat) was once a week for quite a while we had sessions. Awesome sessions, the best of talks, and finally I had found someone who could explain the WHYs. It takes a good psychologist some time to unravel the string called your mind, and my string was a tangled mess, but he got it straightened out. Pat explained everything, how I thought the way I did, why I thought the way I did, why I reacted to situations the way I did, and how I had what he called a "fifties" mentality. Must have been too many "Leave it to Beaver" reruns – heck,

I don't know. Honestly though, being a rigid, somewhat obsessive-compulsive, driven person, once you understand the why, it makes a tremendous difference. If you understand and channel your energy constructively you could write a book, or build a Fortune 500 company, or be a professional athlete – really, anything you desire.

Oh, and the alcohol abuse, yes that, now I had the answer. You see, I am what is called a "problem drinker", and problem drinkers are not addicted in the way an alcoholic is. Frankly, in my own selfish way, I sometimes thought, "Shoot, I wished I did have an addiction problem; then I could get sympathy; then I could blame it on someone or something else and not be accountable for my own problem." Nope, not happening. Own it, Big Boy; be a man, and accept who you are, the good with the bad. Problem drinking is, in a way, more insidious than anything. You can start at any time and at the drop of a hat just take some time off, quit for a while. See, I don't have a problem, I can stop anytime I want. Except when the binge starts, then the obsessiveness kicks in and its hammer city. You may be a happy drunk, you may be a sleepy drunk, you may be an asshole drunk, but you are still a drunk, and that, my friends, is the problem. You see, problem!

Pat asked me once if I was paranoid. I responded emphatically, "NO!" He would continue his probing, "So, do you go out when you drink?" "Well, no," I would respond. He would explain that's the paranoia kicking in, that fear.

Wow, enlightening!

I was the master at hiding, sneaking, and not owning my problem. Hell, I did not have a problem; I could quit anytime!

Yeah, sure I could.

My time with Dr. Long was the best thing I could have done, and to this day I share my experience and time with him with anyone and everyone. I am just a regular guy, who has had his fair share of issues. Sure, mistakes are made; sure, things might have been different. But you see, that's the beauty of life—the past is just that, past. The future is where all of our potential lies in all of us. Change and improvement, it resides in all of us; you just have to want it badly enough.

I believe I owe my life to Dr. Long; as with many of my mentors, he was such a major component in helping me become a better person. His kindness and caring attitude I will always remember. I will never forget our last session when he said, "Tom, our time is done. You are one of the most normal people out there, and you just needed to figure a few things out."

Yes, lightning can strike twice.

> "
> Great discoveries and improvements invariably
> involve the cooperation of many minds. I may
> be given credit for having blazed the trail, but
> when I look at the subsequent developments I
> feel the credit is due to others rather than to
> myself.
>
> ~Alexander Graham Bell
> "

23: PMA- The Power of a Positive Mental Attitude

I once read a book called *Connected*[19], and it really drove home the principles of networks, friends, family and synergy, affiliation, building the network, and how technology can help with re-socialization, incentivize involvement. Networks come in all shapes; it is one of the key premises in this book, from the beginning of print we talked about types. Neurological, social, telephony, internet, marketing— I needed an acronym, something to start this section; I needed my own acronym, but the best I have is PEN, the "Positive Energy Network".

The Positive Energy Network is directly linked to the following behaviors:

- Faith

- Optimism

- Hope

- Integrity

- Initiative

- Courage

- Generosity

- Tolerance

- Tact

- Kindness

- Good sense

All of these are essential to building the network, and they all lead to the strength that is needed to be successful.

My 30 years and two college degrees in the telecom industry always lead me back to technology. Understanding networks and the laws behind the networks are key in our modern times; first there is Moore's Law. The law is named after Intel co-founder Gordon E. Moore, who described the trend in his 1965 paper. The paper noted that the number of components in integrated circuits had doubled every year from the invention of the integrated circuit in 1958 until 1965, and predicted that the trend would continue "for at least ten years". His prediction has proved to be uncannily true, in part because the law is now used in the semiconductor industry to guide long-term planning and to set targets for research and development.

Second is the key to network diffusion, Metcalfe's Law, which states that the value of a telecommunications network is proportional to the square of the number of connected users of the system (n2).

First articulated in this form by George Gilder in 1993, and credited to Robert Metcalfe in regard to Ethernet, Metcalfe's Law was initially presented circa 1980, not in terms of users, but rather of "compatible communicating devices" (for example, fax machines, telephones, etc.). Only recently with the launch of the Internet did this law carry over to users and networks, as its original intent was to describe Ethernet purchases and connections. The law is also very much related to economics and business management, especially with competitive companies looking to merge with one another. You could also use this network metaphor in our friendships, socialization, nervous system… anything, really. I ruminate that all of this is directly related to our belief and faith that we spoke of earlier.

The PEN (Positive Energy Network) is the key to achieving goals, but even more important is its inherent ability to build on the "Law of Attraction".

The "Law of Attraction" is one of the most powerful of all laws, but it does seem to fit what we are trying to accomplish—moving forward in our lives. I have been so extremely fortunate to have attracted mentors, that I had to blend the PEN together with the Law of Attraction because of them. Nothing in this world will boost your positive attitude, your confidence in success, like mentors. And never forget that mentors can be older or younger; age has no bearing. I had to come to grips with my anxiety and feelings of inadequacy (in everything, but especially college); confidence takes time to build, and without my mentors I would never have accomplished the majority of my academic and physical accomplishments.

When I was faced with difficult choices my network of help had to grow, and seeking and finding these people saved my life, like Dr. Long, another of my many friends and mentors.

Ask yourself this: Who in your network could make a positive change in your life, that difference; when you need guidance who can you turn to? It only takes that first effort of outreach to start the process; that is where Metcalfe's Law has bearing, because it is through that first member of your team that you gain the confidence to keep moving forward, and believe me the second mentor is just waiting to help, which leads to the next and to the next. It is the PEN's greatest attribute, and the Law of Attraction will bring these people to you, but you have to make the first move.

The right mentor can change your life forever. Read books and study, but never be afraid to ask; educators love to help, but you have to make the first move.

If you are going to be successful in creating that dynamic life of your dreams, the perpetual Indian summer of your life, you first have to take the faith we have built, coupled with the energy of your belief in yourself, and charge forward. Positive energy attracts like energy (similar energy), like a magnet you will draw upon the energy of the universe and will fuel your engine of success. Many super-successful people have admitted to not being the most talented or gifted, but they had one quality over all others—their positive energy was unstoppable, their positive energy deflected all negatives, and their work ethic was paramount because they believed.

Through adversity lives opportunity, like my college years, the journey to the fitness goals, body building, radio talk show, enlightenment empowering others through mentors and being a protégé myself. It was all due to the PEN.

Focusing on good, on positives in your daily life causes you to attract, like butterflies to flowers, more good, creating a positive feedback loop, a virtuous cycle that gains strength. This loop in effect acts as a force field—remember the Star Trek television show, where the deflector shields would protect the ship; remember that?

Pareto Principle

The Pareto principle (also known as the 80-20 rule, the law of the vital few, and the principle of factor sparsity) states that, for many events, roughly 80% of the effects come from 20% of the causes. This is another academic principle that can have a direct metaphorically related effect in our PEN.

Business-management consultant Joseph M. Juran suggested the principle and named it after Italian economist Vilfredo Pareto, who observed in 1906 that 80% of the land in Italy was owned by 20% of the population; he developed the principle by observing that 20% of the pea pods in his garden contained 80% of the peas. It is a common rule of thumb in business; e.g., 80% of your sales come from 20% of your clients. Laws of economics hold true for our network, that as a barrier to help repel negative energy, 20% of your energy can repel 80% of the destructive behavior.

Feeding the network

Opportunity can be, for example, a goal of doing good deeds for the day.

The windows of opportunity:

- See it (the window)

- Approach it and look through it

- Make your move—jump through (experience), or

- Close it (deny the opportunity)

It really is about the positive energy; think of turning on the light in the refrigerator—you have to open the door first!

24: The bodybuilding show—You have got to be kidding!

If I ever needed a PEN it was when the suggestion to compete in a body-building show occurred. Now let me set the record straight right now—I think deep down every person wants to think they have the body to compete in something like this. I mean, let's be honest, it is flattering to think you could look as solid as some of those people. I do not mean massively gigantic like some of these cats, just symmetrically very strong and fit. I admit it was a bucket list thing that I had. But I was going on 51 years old when this suggestion came around, and this is not normally something that you just decide to do, or is it? In the growing of my PEN (Positive Energy Network), I had become close to Chris Johnson; remember I talked about Chris in the motivation section, and he's been on the talk show, etc. Anyway, as I was building my friendship (it is my opinion that when you build your PEN your relationships with people grow, Law of Attraction, I digress, sorry), it was through Chris that the suggestion to do this show was born.

Skeptical? Oh, yeah. Could I do this? Well, I thought so. So the planning for this event started to grow. I knew that there were several positives that could come from doing this: first and foremost it helped my PEN, because mentors make all the difference and training with a guy like this, learning, becoming friends, would only help with my knowledge curve. Chris is the man and was willing to share; I would have been a fool not to take him up on his offer. Secondly it is the goal of making that large of a commitment. I mean, this is no easy task—doable for sure, but easy? No way. My confidence was in need of a jolt, so once I made up my mind it was balls to the wall, baby. Thirdly I wanted to learn and build credibility and derive content for our website—what a great opportunity. I knew in my heart that this was something that not many people do (actually after I discovered that very few people start competing at this age, I had one competitor and trainer tell me it was "unheard of"). It would help give me not only confidence, but help in building my network, meeting other athletes. But it was a window of opportunity that I had to jump through; networks are like that sometimes—you gotta reach out and extend yourself.

It is true, I found out that once you decide, once you commit, once you make your move and get that brain going (consciously and subconsciously), the refrigerator door opens and the light comes on, if you believe that anything is possible.

I will talk about the prep, the thumbnail-size suit, the eating program, the training twice a day for 16 weeks, parading around on stage in front of 500 people; I have to share this at this point because of my feeling of the PEN; it was a key to fulfilling this goal.

25: Community service, giving back the essence of our country

I had the opportunity to conduct several youth camps while figuring out our business model; it really was an extension of the volunteer coaching Sandy and I did for years, just in a different format. I have and always will believe that group activities are the best form of socialization; you can break down prejudices, make new friends, and have that sense of accountability to your group and yourself. I believe that the boomers have a huge advantage in our life skills to give back our tacit knowledge, and frankly the time is perfect and it is really needed.

The youth fitness camp was really a beta-test that I wanted to conduct along with my colleagues Regie Rieder and Patty Oehmke, and together we came up with a format that I plan on pursuing, along with everything else that I have going on. It was really a basic exercise station, circuit format with limited equipment. That was part of the plan—can you get a bunch of high-schoolers to join in an exercise class without all the fancy bells and whistles? Just basic stuff: jump rope, ladder drills, bouncing balls to develop hand eye coordination, BOSU balance stuff, really simple. Take that run around in stations for an hour and then I incorporated an academic component, where I invited in an adult every week to talk to the kids about life, for no more than half an hour. We conducted this camp at a local inner city high school.

In essence it was a smashing success; the feeling I derived from giving to these young people taught me that the concept of the PEN will work. This was a very mixed group, male and female, freshman to seniors, and most of them did not know each other. I took care of that right from the start by putting these 20 or so kids in a circle and having them shake hands with each other and introduce themselves, and then the old-fashioned football way of white tape with your name on your shirt re-enforced who they were. People like to hear their own names, and I like to be able to motivate by yelling and joking with the kids on a first-name basis. You know what? The system worked. Not only did they all have a better spring season (these were all spring athletes), they had some of the best seasons in a long time. Our baseball boys made it to the Regionals for the first time in over 20 years.

My point with this story has several components. First, the volunteerism aspect of this camp (this was a free camp) far outweighed the same camp we ran for a fee. The fee camp was a hassle and kids did not show up; that was an interesting observation, maybe a testament to our softer young people who don't want to participate when mom and dad pay, but when you have a bunch of inner city kids who don't have squat they show up and work hard and appreciate your time. Secondly, I personally derived a tremendous feeling of satisfaction from this beta-test. Intrinsically I felt better and it helped charge up my PEN and increase the outreach, too.

Frankly, it was a blast.

I hope to continue with this down the road, and I wanted to share this with my boomer brothers and sisters for the simple reason of just thinking about community service. I have done it through my coaching, which is one of my talents, but what are yours? Think about that—our country needs your input and so do our young people. They need you to encourage positive life skills, share your knowledge, become friends with them and help them to succeed. You will be amazed at what can happen when you give freely of yourself and your time.

Community service is the backbone of our great country.

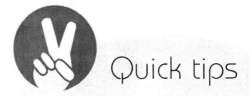 Quick tips

- Your PEN needs constant recharging.

- Try this first thing in the morning—an affirmation; say, "I believe" three times.

- Leave love notes, secret hidden notes to your loved ones.

- Change the ratio of your mental input and positive constructive thoughts; this conditions your RAS.

- Think about your self-esteem, self-image and competence; think positive.

- Love yourself more.

- Just because someone does not recognize your gift does not mean you don't possess it.

26: Solving the NET —The Negative Energy Tornado

Why does the weather man always refer to a forecast as a 30% chance of rain, instead of a 70% chance of sunshine?

The video game culture, work ethic, living in your parents' basement, settling for less, being way too comfortable, play dates and the empty park, just random thoughts about why boomers need to think about outreach; we were not part of the video game generation. Settling for less was not in our gene pool, only getting ahead and busting ass.

Being way too comfortable – no, that is what we have done to our kids; by us working long and hard, we have conditioned our kids to live in the basement until they are 40! And by making this a way to a comfortable life, we have allowed this younger generation to become the first group of people who are projected to live shorter lives than their parents, a first in the modern era. If we allow this to continue, we fuel the NET.

The NET (Negative Energy Tornado), as it grows stronger becomes darker, blocking all light. Its magnetic force holds and grows, pulling more energy into its vortex, gaining strength and absorbing everything and everyone that dares to come close; it is evil. Protect yourself through awareness.

Negative thinking can decrease blood flow to your brain and lessen brain activity; it can cause your heart to beat faster, which increases blood pressure, which leads to many peripheral effects throughout your body. That negative thinking can affect your efforts to lose weight, and counter your motivation to exercise or quit a bad habit, for example smoking. Limiting thoughts we hear in our brain can ruin our lives, and we need to find a way to stop the thoughts. The first step is awareness, the second is to stand up to them, challenging them, and thirdly we need to replace them with positive affirmations and thoughts.

The key to dealing with negative thinking is realizing that we are in charge, the captain of our own ship, and we control the destination of our thoughts and the direction of our life. If you agree with or listen to negative thoughts, then you are putting yourself in the position of limiting your beliefs, which directly affects your faith and behavior. We have to communicate with our negative thoughts and understand them, and recognize them for what they are, because they hold the key to our improvement and change. Think of this: is this thought or behavior helping or hurting me? Am I blocking my goal with fear and planting the seed of self-doubt?

27: The national news—is it only bad news?

I did a non-empirical, non-scientific analysis of the national news television broadcast to try and develop a small sample of data on negativity and ad choice. Here are the results:

- 33 minutes total broadcast recorded

- 26 minutes were programming

- 18.05 minutes were actual news stories (broken into segments, one 13.5 min, two 1.5, three 1.5, four 2.75)

- 8.05 minutes were ads (broken into segments, one 2.0, two 3.2, three 2.45)

Of the news stories, here is the breakdown:

- Earthquake and the Washington Monument

- Congressional Disaster Funding (of which there were ten reported)

- Education Nation—the plight of our eighth graders (Ranked 14th globally, 25th in math skills, and 25% can't read)

- Change of laws in schools—Parents triggering change

- Bad weather

- Satellite crash

- Medal of Honor winner—(first positive story, 1.5 minutes)

- Making a Difference segment, The LEAF program—(second positive story, 2.75 minutes)

Commercials and their breakdown

- Nine health-related:
  - *Omnaris (prescription nasal drug)*
  - *Benefiber*
  - *Centrum vitamins*
  - *Advil*
  - *Alka Seltzer plus*
  - *Aleve*
  - *Ensure*
  - *Benefiber (second)*
  - *Restasis artificial tears (eye drops)*

- Four insurance-related
  - *Allstate*
  - *United Healthcare*
  - *Geico*
  - *Prudential*
- Two food-related
  - *Campbell's soup*
  - *Eggs (I forget the brand)*
- One education-related
  - *University of Phoenix*
- One automobile-related
  - *Honda*
- One investment-related
  - *Fidelity (full disclosure: my 403B is with Fidelity)*
- One local television promo
  - *Ad for the Today show*

Okay, so let's add it up: of the eight stories on this segment of the nightly news (and again, full disclosure: we love NBC and Brian Williams, and we watch NBC every time we watch the national news), 18.05 minutes total, with two stories that were positive in nature taking about four and a half minutes, which roughly equates to 25 percent of this show being positive, which I believe is good comparatively speaking, and if Brian Williams didn't have the Making a Difference piece, since it was almost three minutes long, you can see how that would have changed the ratio.

Of the ads, a full one-third of the show was commercials, of which nine of the total 19 ads were health-related in some form, and four were insurance-related, which gives us roughly like 70%, so this is an illustration of one of our favorite shows, the amount of energy that goes into a program and its content. But this is really nothing new. Negative news sells; drive down the freeway and see a fender-bender and the gawkers, and watch how the neck-turners will stop traffic quickly. It is our conditioning that makes us feel the need to look. It is that need that drives content generators, news, newspapers, and internet bloggers to write about disasters. And it requires the ability to recognize these factors, which we must understand, to look at a negative and somehow turn it around into a positive.

Your positive energy can immediately diffuse the NET; it has illimitable power, which can release us from the darkness and will allow the light of the PEN (Positive Energy Network) to shine through. The stronger your belief in your own ability, the stronger the habit becomes, building an energy field that will engulf your life. Use the law of exchange, and think of the swapping of negative (unproductive) energy and/or behaviors for positive (productive) thinking.

Negative thoughts can occur constantly; here are some to think about:

1. All or nothing

2. Always thinking

3. Focusing on the negative

4. Thinking with your feelings

5. Guilt-beating

6. Labeling

7. Fortune-telling

8. Mindreading

9. Blame

All or nothing, or always or never thinking

If you think about it, very few things in life are this way: all or nothing. If we think this way, looking for this black or white outcome, we are setting ourselves up for disappointment. Words like "always", "never", "everyone", "everything", and "every time" put that limitation on us; it is way too much pressure, and none of us are perfect, so stop. If you have a cheat day with your diet, or you miss one day in the gym—big deal, just get back on the pony. If you find these thoughts occurring try this: replacement thoughts. Instead of "I am never going to get into shape", try "This is a long process and I can do it if I stick with it." Believe me—it works.

Focusing on the negative

As we have talked about, when you are bombarded with negative it tends to permeate your thoughts. Just like Mom said about "we are what we eat", well, we are what we think. Some people cannot focus on the good in anything; that is a learned behavior, and it can change. You just have to decide to flip the switch, smile to yourself and think about how the old you would think and go with the negative reaction, and flip it—think about the positive. We need to train our positive muscle; it takes time and will not happen overnight. I find doing positive affirmations on Facebook to be really helpful for me. Try it—I am amazed at how many people will send me a note when I don't post regularly; it works and it starts your day in the right direction.

Thinking with your feelings

"I feel like... something is wrong!" Is it? Or are you just talking yourself into a situation? Is it, in fact, true? Don't assume. Assumption will spin you into the negativity; get the facts and then make your decision.

Guilt

These are the telltale words: "must", "should", "ought to", "have to"; again, it feeds the tornado. Try this instead: "it is in my best interest", "it would be wise if I", "it supports my overall goals to". Guilt will never be productive, and should be avoided. It will become a barrier to positive results and sabotage your efforts; understand guilt and be stronger than the feeling.

Labeling

Labeling is attaching some made-up phrase, name or condescending term, for example, "loser", "idiot", "moron", "dumbass", "stupid". Don't use these; they feed the tornado and serve absolutely no purpose, and it lumps you into a category of people who think the same way, so break the cycle.

Fortune-telling

Creating a terrible catastrophe in your mind can be one of the worst of our negative thoughts, thinking you just know something terrible is going to happen will open your mind to the inevitable tornado-building monsoon. Predicting the future is a natural and human quality, but be aware of its power to spin backwards and feed the tornado, and think positive and watch what happens.

Mindreading

Never assume anything; the assumption process is probably going to plant a bad seed and grow the weed— just ask if you are wondering about someone's feelings. Try this, "I am getting the feeling from you...", or "Are you mad at me?" Just ask; when in doubt check it out.

Blame

The worst of the worst is blame. How many times have you blamed someone or something for your situation, your position in life, and your status? "It is your fault" is a negative, and kills accountability; stop and own it. Not being honest and having no integrity are problems in our society; it is much easier to blame someone else for a situation, but it does not solve a thing. If there is a problem let's look to resolve the issue logically and intelligently. Blaming is never going to cure anything; is a terrible habit and can ruin your life.

Forward thinking, getting in front of your life, can set the stage for improvement and growth. Everything happens for a purpose, and the pieces to the puzzle of life fit together perfectly. When you believe in these thoughts you'll be amazed at the potential that you have at your disposal. The word "omnipresence" means to be everywhere, and positive energy is omnipresent. The power of positive energy exists in everything; we just need to find it. It is through loving ourselves and education, the enlightenment of knowledge and accountability that diffuses the tornado.

28: Happiness

Dr. John A. Schindler's definition of happiness is, "A state of mind in which our thinking is pleasant a good share of the time." I like it, a lot!

All of us, it does not matter age, race, or creed, we all desire that eternally good feeling in our hearts of happiness. We think better, perform better, feel better (physically and emotionally), and are healthier when we are happy. If you ask people the characteristics of a good life, you will likely hear happiness, health and longevity—the boomers' big three and "Boomers Rock" mantra of QOL.

Happiness is inherent to the human species, and our physical machines; it's what makes us rock.

There have been studies done that state when people are thinking happy, pleasant thoughts that things taste, smell and sound better; that according to Russian psychologist K. Kekcheyev. Dr. William Bates showed and proved that eyesight improved when a person thought about pleasant sights.

Happiness is a state of mind.

When a person realizes that true and lasting happiness is available to anyone and everyone, why would you not want to overcome any weakness to achieve it? Happiness needs to have a strong foundation, a footing like a strong home needs, to withstand the negativity of our world, the aforementioned NET.

So when do you choose happiness? How about right now, this second! This is the key to starting your happiness motor; turn the key, pull the ripcord and make that conscious decision to be happy. Sounds hard, but it isn't. The hardest part is just deciding and believing that you can in fact be happy and live a happy life; happiness is a state of mind, a state to which you must open yourself up, first and foremost, and let it happen. Start your day with a positive thought. Try this: think to yourself when you open your eyes in the morning, "This is going to be a wonderful day, full of happiness and prosperity." Think positive, happy thoughts right from the start of your day. Use the law of attraction, become a happiness magnet, use your PEN to invigorate your thoughts; joy is my partner and love is my heart.

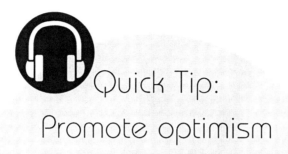

Quick Tip:
Promote optimism

Winners have the ability to fabricate their own optimism. No matter what the circumstance, the happy person will always find a way to see the glass as half full. They know that failure is a type of adversity and through adversity grows opportunity. Those who think in that optimistic thought process can always get the most out of any situation.

I think that sometimes we tend to get things backward, for example, "Be good," we think, "and I will be happy." Or, "If only I were successful, I would be happy," or, "If I were healthier, I would be happy." These are limiting beliefs. Why not think this way, and turn it around? "Be happy—and I will be successful, or healthier, or good to others." It is what you perceive and believe that will carry your thoughts to others and make change possible.

Happiness is not something that is made or warranted. Happiness is not a moral issue; happiness is that feeling, that state of mind, in which we think pleasantly, positively and productively. When you see past the faults and the negativity, happiness becomes one of the keys to removing the power of the NET (Negative Energy Tornado). As Spinoza wrote, "Happiness is not the reward of virtue, but virtue itself; nor do we delight in happiness because we restrain our lusts; but, on the contrary, because we delight in it, therefore are able to restrain them."

> "To live fully, as completely as possible, to be happy…is the true aim and end of life."
> ~Llewelyn Powers

Happiness comes from being and acting unselfishly—not a payback for actions, but as a result of them. I have become so aware of the power of community service and giving freely of one's time. The intrinsic feeling that I received by conducting a free camp for at-risk youth was an overwhelming feeling of happiness, for example, enlightened my heart; I really was shocked.

One of the most pleasant thoughts and feelings, which can lead to happiness, is the feeling of being needed or wanted, that you or your actions are important enough to make that difference to another human being. Boomers, you have a tremendous gift at your disposal: your knowledge and wisdom. Use them or lose them. Don't wait and live for the future, looking forward to being happy or doing those unselfish acts of community service, helping others and waiting for happiness to arrive; be proactive, go get it, be aggressive. Remember that happiness is like the seed of life; it is a mental habit that needs to be planted, cultivated and cared for, so don't wait!

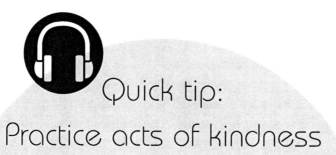

Quick tip:
Practice acts of kindness

Performing an act of kindness can release the brain chemicals serotonin and dopamine (very powerful neurotransmitters, feel-good chemicals). Selflessly assisting someone is a powerful way to feel good about yourself, and acts of kindness will always come back to you. I like to think it is good karma. Acts of kindness can promote a cascading effect, delivering that feel-good chemical, but also encouraging others to respond in positive ways. Acts of kindness are unquestionably a NET diffuser.

It is hard to escape the power of networks; again, as I iterated earlier, it is networks that drive the power of humans. Bell, Metcalfe, Moore, Edison, Einstein, all of these brilliant people had one commonality: they used networks to increase their reach. Happiness is no exception; rather I believe it is directly connected to success.

The famous Framingham Heart study of 1948 developed statistics that measured the spread of happiness through social networks. The researchers examined the relationships of more than 1000 people of the original 12,067 persons in the survey, and found that clustering occurred; happy people cluster with happy people, and unhappy cluster with unhappy—a sort of "misery loves company" scientific analysis. It is possible that happy people might choose each other as friends or be exposed to the same environment that causes them all to be happy at the same time. This phenomenon is described as the "degree of separation", where it is hypothesized that everyone is only separated by six degrees (a friend is one degree, the friend's friend is two, and so on), so in essence happiness and/or unhappiness are closely related due to social networks. The clustering of people with like behavior was statistically documented to also have an effect on earning income, or perhaps evidence leans

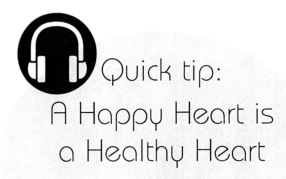

Quick tip: A Happy Heart is a Healthy Heart

A new Columbia University study found that happier people are less likely to have heart attacks, clogged arteries, and other cardiac problems. The researchers used a five-point scale to measure people's happiness and found that for every point increase, heart risks declined by 22 percent.[20]

toward the thought that having happy friends and relatives appears to be a more effective predictor of happiness than earning more money.

Studies have shown that negative factors such as obesity and smoking (unhappy tendencies) tend to spread among networks—fuel for the NET; however, positive factors (happiness) work in just the opposite way—energy for the PEN. In fact, knowing an individual who is happy can produce a 15 percent greater likelihood that you will be happy as well, and there is a nine percent increase in your chances of being happy if one of your friends has a happy friend, a two degree of happiness separation.

So what causes the behavior of someone else (happiness, unhappiness, depression) to affect our mindset? The answer lies in our brain, where there exists what are called mirror neurons. Mirror neurons make humans unique; they give us the unique ability to mimic and react to behavior and are directly linked to our behavior. When you smile at someone, chances are their mirror neurons fire and they smile back; neurologists believe that mirror neurons are the part of our brains that give us the ability to empathize, to feel someone else's issues, mindful insight. If someone is happy and you are directly connected to them, for example in a face-to-face conversation, than your mirror neurons want you to be happy as well.

Happiness is something that we all deserve, and you can have yours; it is just discovering what your compelling "why" is. What is it? What is yours? And lastly, how can we take increasing our own happiness and mix it with making our world a better place? Now that's the question!

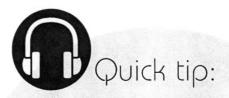

Quick tip:
Nurture social networks and relationships

The happiest people in our world are those who have meaningful, deep relationships; conversely, mortality rates are doubled when we are lonely. Make sure you reach out and decrease the degree of separation—you may save someone's life, and help yourself as well. Networks and outreach are the keys to being happy.

29: Habits

YOU MAKE YOUR HABITS, AND THEN YOUR HABITS MAKE YOU!

Remember how I love to use the planting the seed analogy, "as you sow, so shall you reap"? It means that our lives are created by what we do, not by what we intend. It means that we can harvest only what we plant. And every day you're planting something, so choose wisely.

It has been estimated that ninety percent of our daily lives are habitual, 90%! From the time we wake up until the time our heads hit the pillow, habits form our daily lives.

Over time we develop many sets of firmly entrenched "neural pathways", maps, habits. These paths determine how well every area of our lives function, from our jobs to our personal hygiene—everything. These can be good maps (habits), or bad. We can develop bad posture, and it can become very hard to correct; we can develop self-defeating, Negative Energy Tornado-feeding habits that can inhibit our growth, limit our success, and contribute to our failures.

Sigmund Freud has been quoted as using the term "mental plasticity" to describe a person's capacity for change, and he realized that everyone is different in their own capacity to change, to modify a habit. Freud also observed that a "depletion of plasticity" tended to occur in many older people, leading them to become "unchangeable, fixed, and rigid", which he attributed to a "force of habit." He also wrote, "There are some people, however, who retain this mental plasticity far beyond the usual age-limit, and others lose it very prematurely."

I would like to say once again, it is the "use it or lose it" phenomenon. It is our conscious choice to adapt our unconscious behavior. Whatever habits we currently have ingrained are what are directly attributing to our status in our lives at this moment. If we desire to step up, to reach a higher level of success, then the choice is clear; we must identify, attack, and change self-defeating, negative habits.

Whatever habits we have established, they are a precursor to our behavior and the reason we achieve our current level of outcomes. If we decide we want to create change, to achieve a higher level of behavior, to become a happier, more fulfilled person, we are going to have to identify and then drop some of the self-defeating habits. For example, negative comments, sarcasm, staying up late, not answering e-mail and blowing off responsibilities all need to be switched to more worthwhile productive habits. Complimenting others, setting a stronger and healthier sleep schedule, following through on commitments, and returning e-mails take the fuel away from our negative habits. Remember how I described the NET, and see how the small things can contribute to the brewing tornado of negativity. A lot of times these things start as innocent, very small actions, and then lead into a spiraling out of control lifestyle—stop! Your habits will determine your outcome; successful people do not get to be successful by magic. It is the consistent positive behavior, the PEN-building that takes discipline and will lead to change and reward.

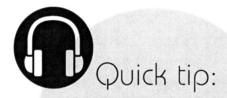

Quick tip:

No better time than the present, take action to develop healthier habits at this instant!

Here is the plan—make a list. Any habitual behavior that you find feeding your NET, write it down, list it out, if it negatively affects your lifestyle, write it down. Request input from your family, your closest friends; get feedback on anything that is annoying or counterproductive and then look for patterns. Here are some of mine, some I have corrected, some are still a work in progress:

- Forgetting someone's name as soon as you are introduced

- Not following through on promises

- Talking too much in a group conversation

- Late night eating

- Missing your children's events

- Eating fast food

- Not sharing your love with others, and actively expressing it

Once we identify the habits, even if it is just one, then try and make a replacement alternative. For example if you want to get more exercise time in, but you just feel you don't have enough time in your day, try this: Go to bed 15 minutes earlier, and get up 10 minutes earlier and stretch; you have a net gain of five minutes of sleep time, and you have added one third of your needed daily exercise time. I have used this method and it works great. You can build on this as you adjust your new schedule, slowly getting up earlier, and not feeling like you have to get up really early.

After six months the getting up a half an hour earlier is no big deal because you slowly adjusted your body clock; a new habit is established, so good for you!

Just imagine if we established two new habits a year, just two—in five years we have 10 new habits and I guarantee you will see a tremendous difference; give it time and stick with the plan—it works! Write down your new goals, those Positive Energy Network-building blocks, put sticky notes on the fridge, post reminders, and keep the energy and the positivity growing—habits take time to establish.

We are creatures of habit. Habits are a function of our subconscious mind. We learned how to ride a bike,

throw a ball, dance, or play an instrument by consciously practicing. Remember the deep practice? It takes
time to establish the tracks. My friend and colleague
from the talk show Dr. Lori Shemeck (she is a psychologist from Texas) called it "making a path in the grass".
I call it snow hill sledding. At that point the automatic
habit action took effect and our subconscious took over.
Sometimes these are referred to as second nature. We
are compulsive beings, so actively choosing good or bad
behaviors are up to us. If you have a deep desire to release yourself from a destructive habit, you are more
than halfway there. When your desire, your compelling
"why" is greater than the habit, you are on your way;
the difficulty of quitting, of making the change is right
in front of you.

I used tobacco for over 17 years. To this day I still
do not know why I started; it is a disgusting habit, and
it became an addiction. Snuff tobacco delivers a potent
punch of nicotine to your system, so even though I never
smoked cigarettes I can empathize with smokers and
their plight in trying to quit. Finally I decided I had to
end this mess, and the cost was just ridiculous, so I substituted two things to get over this addiction: the money
that I had in my pocket and cinnamon toothpicks. You
know what? After all those years I broke that disgusting spitting gooey habit, and thank God, because the
health issues that go along with this stuff is awful; I
count my blessing every day. It was really hard, but I
made up my mind and that was that.

Here are the stages involved with breaking a habit:

1. *Early stage*—"The first few days are always the
   most difficult. Old habits are hard to break. The
   mental process must be on guard continually to
   provide the right action."

2. *Middle stage*—"The moment good habits begin to take root, options open that bring on new challenges. New habits are formed that will be either good or bad. The good news is: 'Like begets like.' The more right choices and habits you develop, the more likely good habits will be formed."

3. *Later stage*—"Complacency can become the enemy. We all know of incidents where someone (perhaps us) successfully lost weight, only to fall back into old eating habits and gain it back."

Habitual behavior change is tough because it takes time, and therein lies the problem. We have become so conditioned to instantaneous gratification, to a quick fix, and a silver bullet that long term is a tough sell. My answer to that is small steps. Overnight is not going to solve anything, and habits take time to begin *and* end. The thrill of victory comes long after your decision is made, and by that time your habit is so ingrained that you forget it is a habit, which is why it is important to think about where we have come from and where we are now. Weight Watchers, Alcoholics Anonymous, and stop-smoking clinics are examples of behavior modification groups that use the power of socialization and peer pressure to make us accountable, to help us achieve our goals and change our habits. Tell people what you are working toward, your goal, be excited about your plan, and get pumped up; the embarrassment of failure can be a strong motivator. If there is no support group, build one; use your family, be a rallying point, lead! Use the vision board and message board examples to change your limiting beliefs, post pictures and make notes and splash them everywhere; your subconscious needs the reinforcement, so make the conscious decision and move on it.

Lastly, remember that habits are thousands of times more powerful than wishes or dreams, so if you want it—go get it!

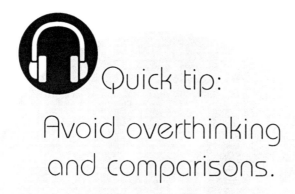

Quick tip:
Avoid overthinking
and comparisons.

Comparing yourself to someone else can be destructive; social comparisons do not come from the PEN—they are components of the NET. If you feel compelled to compare, think about the old you and be happy about progress; love yourself.

> *No passion so effec-
> tively robs the mind of
> all its powers of acting
> and reasoning as fear.*
>
> ~Edmund Burke

30: Fear

Fear is that insidious ingredient of the NET that can hurt all of our efforts to change and improve. Remember how I talked about the fear of that first class way back in 2000, the one with the 400 really smart young people who were all looking at the older guy in the front? I think I described it as terror, but in essence it was simply fear, fear of the unknown, and that's where the rub is—being ill-prepared or not having the right or relevant information or plainly not being educated enough. It's a perfect recipe to build the anxiety that surrounds the fear. It does not know—again, unknown—but not insurmountable, not at all. Fear is a feeling, worrying about looking bad in front of a group, because as we all know, everyone is looking at ME, right? How about the memory of a past relationship that clouds the desire to find a new relationship, a fear of failing, again; hey, I have been there also, a failed marriage, and "oh, poor me" attitude, and what it came down to for me was the fear of being hurt, again, and therefore sitting on the sideline. You might be afraid that you may lose what little money you have saved, and are therefore unable to pull the trigger on that next deal, or new venture. Fear can paralyze us.

Speaking of fear, check this out:

Quick story on Bodybuilding

When I was standing off stage just before the body-building contest in 2010, standing there in something smaller than my underwear, spray tanned like some freak, and greased up like a clown getting ready to do my individual routine, I was hyperventilating with fear. Not only was I a rookie at almost 51 years old, and therefore completely inexperienced in this whole thing, but I could not make up my mind on the routine, and I had like two minutes before I went on stage in front of over 500 people. Now granted I had practiced this at home for a couple of months, and this basically was a 90-second routine to a song of your choice, so I knew the music cold, and I had two routines that I had practiced: the conservative, "just go out there get it over with" standard bodybuilder flex routine (I know, I know, people hear about this and think, "Huh?" It was a goal, a bucket list thing), and the much more energized kind of, in my mind, the Michael Jackson dance routine (yes, I know, kind of bizarre).

When it was my turn, I swear that as I walked out on that stage I still had no idea which one to do, so when the music started I let my fear go. What the hell—I was on the stage all gooped up and had worked like a dog for the past four months getting ready for this, so let's go. So I did the dance routine.

Well, let's say it was a hit; the dance routine went into autopilot, the crowd loved it because it was so different, and it was over in like a blink of an eye.

To this day I have had to watch the video of this thing to remember the routine, because when my fear went out the window it was like a different person, an out of body thing and I could not remember any of it when I came off stage, none of it, and everyone told me how great it was. WOW! Letting my fear paralyze me would have been unacceptable; that was it, no way was I going to chicken out on this one, and to this day it is the confidence that gained from doing something so outrageous that fuels my desire to build out the next phase of my life.

Do not let the fear of failure become a roadblock to your achievement. You can do it; you can do anything if you work hard enough to achieve that goal—I promise you that.

You can see the video at http://www.youtube.com/watch?v=_4y64j6FjH4

Psychologists use this acronym:

Fantasized

Experiences

Appearing

Real

Try this simple technique to alleviate anxiety: diaphragmatic breathing. It takes practice, but think of like this: Close your eyes and focus on your upper abdomen, breathe slowly and deeply not from your upper chest but your upper gut, focus, slowly. From a physical perspective it takes only three conscious diaphragmatic breaths to reduce our blood pressure and pulse rate, to rid our blood of lactate, and to generate the alpha brain waves, which can bring you into your "Zone". How many breaths do we take a day? Approximately 20,000. Yes, twenty thousand. So focusing on three, consciously focusing, can make for a tremendous stress and anxiety release. Practice this skill—it works.

"If you don't manage your money, your money will manage you!"

~Dr. Norman Vincent Peale

As boomers we have many things that we fear, and I believe the first is financial fears and the stress that goes hand in hand with that. So let's talk about financial stress and fear. I know it bugs me. Financial wherewithal—as boomers we just have to have it!

On the radio show "Boomers Rock" I specifically started a segment on financial fitness, knowing full well that without some kind of financial fitness knowledge, talking about our situations, looking at what is happening with the Federal Government and our states' budgets, I would be doing us all a disservice. Probably the biggest stress factor facing us boomers involves financial issues. Entitlement programs are being chopped, our equity in our homes is a mess, insurance programs – well, who knows? And on and on. So when the going got tough I figured it was time to get busy.

Remember what I say on the talk show:

"Through adversity grows opportunity."

People fail to develop financial independence because they fail to develop a winning mentality; I know I did for the longest time. Until becoming educated and associating with someone with great financial common sense, I was a mess. Thank God I married Sandy! The stresses of financial difficulties invariably will catch up to those who allow their spending to come before their common sense. It is a conditional disorder that has completely overwhelmed our society. But like sugar or salt, great when used sparingly, easy credit and this "spend now, pay later" conditioning is a terrible cancer on our lives.

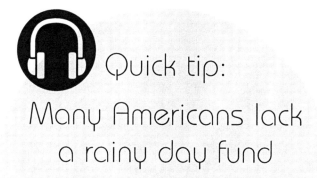

Quick tip:

Many Americans lack a rainy day fund

47% is the percentage of Americans (according to Time Magazine) who said their household couldn't come up with $2,000.00 in 30 days without selling some possessions.

Here are six suggestions to help with financial fear:

1. Procrastination is caused by poor spending habits learned in our earlier years. The boom years are over, and unless you want to continue working full-time the rest of your life, quit waiting around and get busy tidying up your financial house.

2. Avoid poor goal-setting; in other words have a clue on the direction you want your life to move into. If something comes up and derails your goals, don't throw your hands up and cry about it—get off the canvas, wipe the sweat out of your eyes and get busy.

3. Become educated. Our biggest problem in our society is the lack of financial education. Hey, been on that train myself, I admit it; however, just because they did not teach it in college, on the job or wherever, doesn't mean you shouldn't make an effort to become educated. It's your money, right? And there are plenty of self-help books out there, so go buy one. I suggest Dave Ramsey's *The Total Money Makeover*. Dave has great straightforward advice and does not pull any punches.

4. Tax law, CPAs and working the system. I don't ever want to imply, advise, or joke around about tax issues, hardly. The one thing I always said when we started GRT Fitness and Boomers Rock Media was I DO NOT want issues down the road with the government, ever. The IRS is an agency not to be played with, so respect the rules. Now that being said, having a professional who looks out for your best interest is huge, but again— learn the rules and play by them.

5. Buy the right kind of insurance—life, health, auto and property. Having an agent who works for you, and I don't mean some fictitious person on the Internet, is huge.

6. Think like a winner! PMA, (positive mental attitude), persistence, self-discipline, being psychologically in the game makes all the difference. There is no reason we cannot all budget our efforts to maximize our ROI (return on investment). Remember, this book is all about QOL!

Stress, and the accompanying fear, are major players in our lives. Boomers need to use their knowledge and experience to laugh off the small stuff. I think this is where we have a tremendous advantage moving forward in the next 10 to 40 years—the old saying, "Been there, done that" ring a bell to anyone?

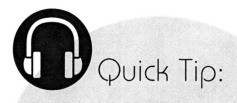

Quick Tip:
Get your computer
skills up to snuff!

According to the employment firm Experience.com, 88% of entry-level positions are now ONLY listed online!

The more you learn to deal with stress, turning the stressor into a positive, the more likely you will continue to get better at your skill. Use it or lose it—sound familiar? Positive and negative energy surround us constantly, distress adds to the negative and the law of attraction will kick in and do its thing—that is, attract like energy. So in essence, the chain reaction is always in place. Optimism builds the positives and pessimism, the negatives. It's a tricky balance, but accepting that the law of attraction is always working, and understanding its power, can help you make better decisions, alleviating distress.

Regardless of what happens, avoid dwelling on "what might have been"; it is probably in our best interest to let it pass. Learning from experiences is the first step to being in control, and that is what we need to focus on. Worrying about coulda, woulda, shouldas is just is a waste of energy. Worrying robs you of your ability to make decisions based on facts, and perpetuates itself as stress and negative energy. See how the vicious cycle starts to spin!

Herbert Benson, M.D., is the Director Emeritus of the Benson-Henry Institute (BHI), and Mind/Body Medical Institute Associate Professor of Medicine, Harvard Medical School. Dr. Benson has authored or co-authored over 180 scientific publications and 12 books. His *The Relaxation Response* was a pioneer in the introduction of the positive effects of meditation, and 10 years later he added another component: "the faith factor". Dr. Benson has made a case for having a strong belief in something; exercise, religion, or just believing in yourself can measurably alleviate anxiety and help manage tension, lower cholesterol and pain levels, and help with insomnia—and of course all of these factors relate to lowering stress.

Dr. Benson is a strong believer in faith and the strong benefits to a person's health and wellness, and that just believing, having faith in yourself or something of a higher spiritual order, can lead to blocking actions of the nervous system that cause stress, tension and sleep issues, all through the holistic measures and not being dependent on drugs.

"If you truly believe in your personal philosophy or religious faith-if you are committed, mind and soul, to your world view-you may well be capable of achieving remarkable feats of mind and body that many only speculate about," Benson wrote[21].

Stress and its accompanying health issues penetrate all levels of our society; it is those who have the outlets, the mechanics to relieve the pressure, who can effectively deal with daily stressors. In our very high-octane society, the instantaneous networked flat world we all exist in, relief is something that should be cherished. Planning for and realizing the need, and providing our bodies with the relaxation we need, must be emphasized.

31: Love

Love is as love does; we choose to share ourselves in love—it is an act of will, pure.

Huey Lewis has some great tunes; I have 37 of them on my iPod, including his Greatest Hits, which is by far a smash great album. This morning, as I finished my work in the lab (er, basement gym), I just happened to flip through the tunes and, BAM, pull out Huey. That in itself is not a huge deal; however, in doing all of my brain readings, material gathering, compiling great information and becoming smarter, I guess I had entered the "Zone", the endorphin zone, and Huey got me thinking, so here are the thoughts, and yes, I think this will make it into the book.

Huey says in his love song, "The power of love is a curious thing," that's for sure.

Powerful stuff no doubt, and a great tune, by the way. Love is an emotion that we all need to have, to experience, and that's why I had to include this in the behavior section of the book. Love is way too large a topic to be truly understood, and for the purpose of this book it really is a simplistic view; however, because it holds so much potential for self-improvement, it is important to talk about. Love involves choice—we chose that person, or thing, to love—and it is an act of will. Love begins with self-sacrifice; read on to see an example of such sacrifice.

When I was in the hospital in April of '08 with that serious illness I spoke about earlier, and before I had a clue as to what was going on, the doctors apparently thought I had something really bad because after one day in the regular ward of the hospital I was shipped over to the "Special Place", the isolation ward. Hmm, since I have always been healthy I certainly had no clue as to why this would happen; however, when the nurses and doctors have to put on the spacesuits to treat you something in the mind tells you, "OH OH, something is not good, this is really not good."

I probably should have thought something was up when my brother had visited me three times that previous day, and if I had looked in the mirror I would have known why, I looked reallllly bad. Anyway—this isolation ward thing, this "special" place had me wondering, again being sick for the first time ever I am more wondering, but still not getting it; being sick will do that to you. I finally had to ask, "What the hell is up with this?" and I got the "precautionary" answer. For what?

Tuberculosis

Ever had that "Oh, shit" feeling?

Now you start thinking about all the little things, like for example, dying. Damn, 48 years old and this could be it – well, that really sucks. Now it's time to start fighting, 'cause I am way too young for this stuff, but unfortunately my body was in no shape to do much fighting.

Let me tell you, and this is the purpose of this little detour, Sandy was the only person, the only one, NOT to put on the suit; and that, my friends, is love. Without her and her love, who knows what would have happened. She knew I would be ok, but that was really risky for her, but a blessing for me because through her confidence I came out of the whole mess ok.

Balls of steel, that blonde woman has, and I am damn glad to have her.

Love is such a strong emotion, and has many depths. The one thing that I always close the show with is this:

> **"To share love with others, you must love yourself first."**

It takes great strength to love, to put yourself out there, to be vulnerable and to understand that you must love yourself, be willing to make the sacrifices necessary to live an enabled and empowered life. If you love and truly love, with no strings attached, no ulterior motives, for the pureness of what it is, then no one and nothing can hurt you; true love is the protector of all human beings.

The more you choose to have a loving attitude, that positive mental attitude, that sense of purpose, understanding the potential of what you and your inner being are capable of, the closer you become to finding that magic. You will appreciate all that surrounds you, and your positive attitude will enable your body to defend itself against the negativity in life. Visualize that perfect body, that healthy relationship, that perfect family; think loving thoughts to all who enter your life, and the power of your love will win over everything. Love is power like no other; it conquers all and does soothe those savages who live in our world.

Life is what happens to you when you are making other plans.

Love the opposites in your life, the objects that cause you the most anguish, because they are what you may be lacking in your life, or they remind you of things you think you want. Forget that wanting, take that place in your heart and turn it around; make it a place for sharing and giving, a place for helping others, because it will be through this that you will be led to that better place in your life.

Genuine love will involve and is given to commitment and thoughtful wisdom. People give of themselves in an action of commitment to who or what they love, be it self-improvement, a hobby or mentorship of others; loving something is work and discipline. The focus of such work is the attention that you will need to devote to that person or thing you love. Listen to your inner being, listen to your spouse, focus on the task at hand and continue to improve; constant work toward a loving outcome and goal is rewarding and doable. Committing yourself is the foundation of any loving relationship, and thought it may not guarantee success, because in life there are no guarantees, you can give yourself the best odds of creating a successful outcome by understanding that the will to commit to your goal is a primary requisite to success. That and being a disciplined, passionate driver to your quest will give you the chance to realize what you are trying to achieve and lead yourself into that place where you can have the QOL we all so desperately desire.

Here is a suggestion, and it works like a charm, is really easy and does not cost a cent; it's called ambush notes. These are quick notes to the ones you love; just writing a quick note can change a person's perspective for the whole day. Such a small gesture can make such an incredible difference in their outlook—it's the gift that does not cost a thing and means so much. Sandy saves all of my ambush notes—all of them!

32: Enthusiasm

One of the most important of all human qualities is the ability to be enthusiastic; it wins over people, can sell a car, pump up a team, or make us a winner! Enthusiasm is contagious; it is one of the shining examples and components of the PEN; it can take a tough situation and make it very doable. Any person who exhibits controlled enthusiasm is normally welcome in any situation; it exudes positive energy. Have you ever been in a situation where the person is enthusiastic about their commitment, their goal, and their ambition? It makes you just want to know more, learn and improve.

One of my key mentors in college was Professor Tom Muth. His enthusiasm to teach, his approachable demeanor, and his gregarious attitude made him a magnet for students; his classes were always packed. I lucked out when I took my first class with Professor Muth (he asked me later in our relationship to call him by his first name), but I just always revered him so much I always referred to him as "Professor Muth".

I did not know his reputation before I enrolled; another gift from God on this one—he changed my life!

The first class I had was what is called a "policy class", a 300-level (undergraduate junior level) course. Professor Muth was not only a Ph.D., but also a J.D., basically a really sharp academic and lawyer; you could say he knew his stuff. I had been back in school for a couple of years by now, so I had learned the lessons of NEVER taking anything for granted, NEVER! (Did I impress the never?)

Again sitting in the front row (and by the way, statistically speaking, students who sit in the front score better on average), I did not have a clue as to what to think of this guy; he spent the first class telling and showing us how to make a card with our name on it—I mean very specifically showing us. You see, it was his way of getting you to become detail oriented, to listen and to follow very specific directions. I had a feeling this guy did not play around; he specifically wanted a certain size font, and a certain type of card stock, and printed landscape style, and he demanded perfection.

His enthusiasm to the class, the energy this older professor brought was unbelievable. He had me hooked the first day I met him.

To say TC-310 was a bitch would be an understatement. The amount of time that went into our weekly assignments was incredible; this was a three-credit course and I was spending 20-30 hours a week on it. I loved it and it was all because of him, because the coursework, policy, can be pretty dry – no, more like borderline awful. Great teachers make awful material great to learn, always remember that!

The energy he brought to this course made you want to work hard; that's what enthusiasm does—it permeates your soul and even the worst of the worst becomes interesting and enjoyable.

I said this earlier, please allow me to reiterate-When you start a class, any class, always start strong; never get lulled into this false sense of security, but rather attack the work from the beginning. That is the benefit we as boomers have over traditional students, that intrinsic work ethic, and that is the quality we need to share with them, guiding and mentoring. When you get going in that course, sit in the front, engage the instructor, teacher or professor, show your desire to learn, your enthusiasm for life and demand the best from yourself. Never go into any class with an eye closed so to speak; be ready right from the beginning.

I was always afraid in the beginning of holding back my enthusiasm. I did not want to stick out and be the old guy in the front always talking; that is a mistake—just be judicious with your questions and points and try

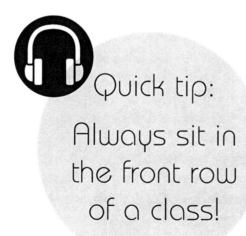

Quick tip:
Always sit in
the front row
of a class!

and engage others in the conversation. No one appreciates someone who dominates the conversation and/or lecture; in this course there were over 150 students, and they paid tuition also. So be aware and respectful of your classmates, but don't be afraid to speak up, too.

As I spoke about earlier, fear can undermine your enthusiasm; be aware, and keep your guard up. Fear can motivate, and it can educate—just learn to use it, and as you overcome and understand the concepts your confidence in yourself will grow and your enthusiasm will blossom. Others have gone through this, many others; it is okay to have feelings of doubt, and it is normal in new situations to be apprehensive, but don't let apprehension and lack of knowledge become a fear that steals your enthusiasm.

> "Aim for the moon. If you miss, you may hit a star."
>
> ~W. Clement Stone

In his book *Believe and Achieve* ("Believe and Achieve", W. Clement Stone, Avon Books, 1991), W. Clement Stone writes extensively about enthusiasm. He points out, "There is a difference between having enthusiasm and being enthusiastic." He also stated that, "enthusiasm is a positive mental attitude-an '*internal*' impelling force of intense emotion, a power compelling creation or expression. It always implies an objective or cause that is pursued with devotion."

However, being enthusiastic is "an impelling '*external*' expression of action. When you act enthusiastically, you accentuate the power of suggestion and autosuggestion. A little difference that makes the big difference is '*attitude*'—especially where enthusiasm is concerned."

If you blend enthusiasm with your work, your work will seem effortless, even fun, key components to our making the "Indian summer" of our lives incredibly exciting. You have more than likely experienced enthusiasm at your job and saw its effect on your co-workers; it is magical how it can build energy. They can become more animated, they feel the energy, the intensity, you can hear it in their voices, and enthusiasm builds through our intrinsic ability to tap into our "mirror neurons".

Mirror neurons

When you see someone stub their toe, you feel the pain; when a baby smiles, you understand the feeling; when a crowd of football fans is overjoyed, you understand and feel the excitement. The enthusiasm, all of these and much more, are caused by mirror neurons. Specialized brain cells that allow humans to be the most wonderful of all creatures, our ability to feel another's pain, or to empathize—these are our mirror neurons. Mirror neurons are an extraordinary type of brain cell, unique to humans, and their abilities need to be understood and exploited to reach the levels of happiness and success, our QOL, that so many desire and deserve.

The sharing of our emotional connections, the outreach, the teaching and of course the learning, are all components of our lives. The ability of our brain to understand and to "feel" someone else's happiness or needs is what drives our enthusiasm to live. It is what makes us so uniquely "human". Being self-aware and in touch with our emotions, reaching deep and feeding our enthusiasm can be read (see mirror neurons), or perceived by others; it feeds the PEN, it enables our happiness, and it empowers others. Mirror neurons give us all the awesome ability to feel someone's love, happiness, and achievements, all through observation.

The possibilities are endless: ESP, self-awareness, learning, duplicating and imitating, or simply helping us become better humans. Enthusiasm for what you love to do can be perceived by others, as we all have "Mirror Neurons".

Never forget, never underestimate, and never give up; life is too precious to underestimate, so live your life like there is no tomorrow, and watch the magic!

Catalyst

I have always been a huge fan of the film "Pay It Forward", starring Kevin Spacey, Helen Hunt, and child actor Haley Joel Osment. Filmed in 2000, the film depicts young Haley as junior high student Trevor McKinney, troubled by his mother's (Helen Hunt) alcoholism and fears of his abusive but absent father, a dysfunctional family similar to many in our society today.

Dysfunction, alcohol abuse, societal misunderstanding, hmmmm... I think I know why I loved the film— parallels to my own life, fall and rise, perhaps?

Digressing once again—sorry!

Trevor is caught up by an intriguing homework assignment from his new social studies teacher, Mr. Simonet (Kevin Spacey). The assignment: think of something to change the world and put it into action. Great stuff, and a tear-jerker for sure; I love this catalyst analogy!

Meanwhile, back on the ranch

Trevor decides on the notion of paying a favor not back, but forward--repaying good deeds not with payback, but with pay forward: new good deeds done to three new people. Trevor's efforts to make good on his idea bring a revolution of sorts, not only in the lives of himself, his mother and his physically and emotionally scarred teacher, but also in those of an ever-widening circle of people completely unknown to him.

His actions lead to an exciting climax, which if you have not seen this film I won't ruin it for you. Suffice to say it is a huge favorite of mine and a classic in my book. I recommend this film not only for the simple fact that it is awesome, but I have shared this story with many friends, trying to illustrate how out of nowhere someone, something, an event can change your life—a catalyst.

Oh, and let the kids watch this one; it may be getting a little bit long in the tooth but it is worth sitting and watching with the kids for sure.

Left to our own devices we go along in a pretty stable mindset. But when we get a clear cue, a message that sends a spark, then boing—we respond. It is that clear clue, that "BOING" effect (remember I was raised on Bugs Bunny cartoons), that we need to make the behavioral change.

Remember how we talked about my epiphany? That triggering mechanism to make someone have the proverbial BOING effect—what people really need (rather than almost dying) is an igniter, the spark to make that first step. From there the momentum starts; it's the flywheel theory—just keep leaning on the stone, pushing with all of your might.

Once the catalyst is introduced, it's magic!

Several years ago while I was still in Graduate school a thought occurred to me while I trained at the gym. You could say this was a catalyst for me in a way, a catalyst which led to much of what I am writing in this book. I regularly saw the same students and faculty working out and training, and I wondered how successful all of these regulars were in their school work or their jobs. I introduced myself and conducted an informal survey.

The bottom line was that virtually all of the regulars, those damn hard workers, all were overachievers. Perhaps it triggered my desire to know more.

What makes people tick? How do you find that trigger, what makes you get off the couch and put down the Doritos? I can tell you that intrinsic love for your effort, whatever floats your proverbial boat, is a trigger. That following through, that keeping the blood flowing, that feeling good about yourself feeds the beast and keeps you looking forward in life. It could be your skinny jeans, or it could be your love for fresh air—it makes no difference.

Do catalysts occur in other people's lives? Can this phenomenon be captured and applied to events to help us trigger positive behaviors? Behavioral shifts that can lead to improving our QOL require us to actively see the process; it is the explosion of possibility that we all must embrace.

I love the thought of catalysts, of meeting people who motivate, and it's probably why I do what I do; intrinsically, I derive my own pleasure from seeing others turn the corner, and by sharing my story, I hope to trigger something in others. If it works for me, it certainly can for you.

Never regret your actions, and always "Pay it Forward!"

Part 2:

FOOD (60%)

Now the fun begins, as we head into the real meat and potatoes of what makes us fuel up and stay healthy, our nutrition, the food factor. Funny that I should word it that way, "meat and potatoes", since we really do not eat all that much of either anymore.

33: Diet Spelled Backwards is Teid

The concept of *a diet* is nonsense. Americans go on diets the way that the French surrender in battle; i.e., constantly, and with the mistaken belief that soon all their problems will go away. But it doesn't solve our basic problem, which is that we absolutely must eat to live. We must eat quality food for our minds and bodies to thrive. However, many forces conspire against us. The industrial-agriculture complex that provides ample food, the fast-food industry that calls out to us seductively to eat their special recipes, and, most damning of all, our own brains that are wired to crave nutrition when offered just in case we need it later on.

The diets we start are like the Maginot line, easily defeated with a side trip through Belgium where, by the way, you can get an oversized Belgian waffle with strawberry sauce and whipped cream, as I'm sure the Germans did on their way to Paris.

Diet crazes, unfortunately, have become ridiculous, riddled with gimmicks to attract attention, and may, in fact, work for certain people because it resonates with their own preconceived notions of eating, nutrition, social settings, and access to food. But even when a gimmick-riddled diet works, our notions of eating, nutrition change. Our social settings shift with friends, the seasons, jobs, and family activities. Fads and advertising may alter our access to nutrition in such a way that the diet's gimmick is defeated.

Diets, in the long run, make as much sense as the nonsensical word *tied*. So how do we make sense of nutrition?

Thinking About Food

I am convinced that inside my brain, somewhere, there lives a gremlin of sorts. We could call it Ghrelin (but that will actually be discussed shortly). Ghrelin is the hunger hormone that sends out the attack signal to your brain that it's time to eat. No, my gremlin that lurks in my brain is a group of synapses that are the ice cream factor. My kryptonite, ice cream, is my absolute Achilles heel. Which actually is okay, and I like to talk about it; it is by understanding the whole behavioral thing that we are able to make improvements in our food consumption.

I have battled with being slightly and even very over-weight my whole life; I can empathize with people who have had this issue. My numbers, weight, cholesterol, blood pressure, sugar have always been borderline high, always. The rollercoaster of being heavy and then not – well, I've been through it all. Did you know that fat cells just go dormant? They shrink down when you lose weight, but balloon up when needed. It's a fact!

When I quit drinking I dropped a ton, all of those empty calories going away really helped, and I started to believe in the "Body for Life" mindset; things were better. But it eventually crept back on, and just like everyone else, I really felt like it was just me being me, chubby, darn dormant fat cells. What I needed was education; I did not have all of the factors, and it wasn't until after the pneumonia (2008, I was 48 at that point), that the epiphany truly rang through.

My time had arrived; I just did not know it, not yet.

Now let me say right here and now that I do not like the word "diet"; I believe we are conditioned to know this word as the silver bullet to all weight issues. Class reunion? Go on a diet. Wedding in the family? Go on a diet. Vacation looming, swimsuit season, fit into that new outfit? Diet, diet, diet. It is the fix-all be-all for weight loss, so what is the problem? Here is my take, a little bit of information

The Cold Truth about the Diet Industry in America

Americans are dieting at the highest rate in history.

20-24% of American men and 33-40% of American women are actively dieting to lose weight.

57% of US women are now dieting according to a national telephone survey.

The diet industry is a multi-billion dollar industry. Over the past twenty years, the diet industry has tripled its gross annual income to approximately $60 billion.

Girls who diet frequently are 12 times as likely to binge as girls who don't diet.

Over one-half of teenage girls and nearly one-third of teenage boys use unhealthy weight-control behaviors (skipping meals, fasting, smoking cigarettes, vomiting and taking laxatives).

Current Diet Mentality of Americans...That is False

It is impossible to be fit AND fat at the same time.

All large people MUST lose weight in order to improve their health and fitness level.

All large people are in poor health.

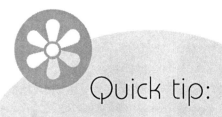

Quick tip:

Something to think about

Only live food that has grown on this planet is suitable for our bodies to transfer the energy and sustenance we need. As science writer Lyall Watson points out in Gifts of Unknown Things, "We did not come into this world. We came out of it, like buds out of branches and butterflies out of cocoons. We are natural products of this earth, and if we turn out to be intelligent beings, then it can only be because we are fruits of an intelligent Earth."

Everyone can lose weight IF they just follow the proper diet and regular exercise program.

The main reason people regain lost weight is THEIR failure to comply with prescribed diets or make long-term commitments to weight loss.

Points derived from the University of New Hampshire[22].

In the beginning

My issue with diets, diet plans, and pseudo-diets is the finiteness of the whole concept, the beginning and the end. I was on the roller-coaster of fitness and weight loss my entire life. Would you like to know my answer? It was education!

I just never put the pieces together, probably like you and many others, I am sure. It wasn't until 2008, and then everything changed. Everything worked.

Let's call it an eating plan, because that is what it is; it is a lifestyle change, not a finite diet but a life-long decision to learn and come to grips with our own gremlins. It is a daily journey, a lifestyle, and it is very simple and doable.

Doctors and economists refer to this term, "opportunity cost", the cost of doing something rather than doing something else; finding your way and changing is the opportunity cost versus not doing anything and hammering chips while you lose your QOL sitting on the couch.

Our opportunity cost of feeling better is directly related to making accountable decisions.

So what is your opportunity cost of not getting off the couch? To not utilizing your skills, sharing knowledge, regaining or losing your QOL—what is it? I will tell you: it is your QOL, and that is too important to let slip away. Together we all make a difference; together we all can share the energy of change.

Balancing this with your ability to do outreach and help others by leading change starts a movement and tips the economies of scale and scope in your favor. It increases your chances of living a longer, healthier life. Now we are getting somewhere; our time is now.

Not doing something positive is a potential for loss and feeds the NET (Negative Energy Tornado); screw that—I want the socialization of the PEN (Positive Energy Network) and the example, that intrinsic feeling of knowing that I helped myself, but also helped others by setting the example and sharing my quest. People need examples and they want to get better!

So what I decided to do, and in the relationship of this book was to share the knowledge in the most concise way I could, is list it out, because frankly it is not rocket science, but it does take some accepting of new thoughts and breaking of those bad habits.

The whole list is in the "Grimoire" section, part four of our book where there is in detailed lists, program, and definitions, the whole package. I separated everything to make it easier to search, and make it a better read. There you will find the complete detailed eating plan, the components and their definitions, and key neurological chemicals and hormones clearly defined.

Moving on

I would like to thank a key person, a good friend, and recommend his book. It incorporates what I have done, which Sandy and I both started to follow.

Chris Johnson[23] is a person I mentioned early in the book, and I want to again thank him for everything he has done as far as encouragement and knowledge. It was through his mentoring that we were able to make the changes, and he was the first person to explain the science behind the nutrition.

His book *Nutrition*, from his "On Target Living" series is a great place to get started on the educational side of weight loss. It is comprehensive and very readable, so I would encourage all of you to pick it up. What I want to share in this section of this book is the synthesizing of what we learned, and the system that we continue to follow, most of which we learned from Chris.

The journey really got rolling in the summer of 2009, several months before the prep for the body-building show. Sandy and I attended a book-signing of Chris's and that is when I befriended him, really on the impetus of learning more about personal training and the business side of the wellness industry.

I have to throw some love to my buddy Regie Rieder for that one; he suggested attending the book-signing where Sandy and I met Chris.

I was reading Paul Zane Pilzer's *The Wellness Revolution*[24] (an awesome read, and one I highly recommend). It was that book, upon finishing grad school, which was my first read. It was this book that was one of my catalysts to moving into that next phase.

Remember I talk about spirituality and the wind blowing our sail into a new place—this book started the wind howling!

As I have stated many times, one thing I learned from Chris, probably THE most important step, is the understanding of the concept of small steps, baby steps, and the act of just making the incremental change. You see, this is where these diets fail—it is the suddenness, the radicalness that dooms us, and what keeps the diet industry making billions.

So here is the plan. I want to list all of my daily activities, the timing, the foods, the supplements, the how and the why, the whole thing, and keep it simple and easy to follow.

> It is very much in the interest
> of the food industry to exacer-
> bate our anxieties about what
> to eat, the better to then to as-
> suage them with new products.
>
> ~Michael Pollen, Author:
> "Omnivores' Dilemma"

34: Hybrid Mediter- ranean Eating Plan—The "HyMEP"

I want to share the things that I used to eat and drink, and how the prepping for the bodybuilding show led to our Hybrid Mediterranean Eating Plan (HyMEP). I mean, I had no idea that we were actually following the Mediterranean plan. Frankly I had never heard of it, but in becoming more educated I realized we had inadvertently stumbled upon our own version of something that has been around for a long time and, frankly, has been very successful. If it has worked for us, it certainly can work for anyone.

I can only tell you how I feel, what has been an almost solid four years of success, and how our QOL has changed and improved; it is amazing.

The HyMEP is consistent with several guidelines. I don't want to call anything a rule—that lends itself to the proverbial "DIET" mindset. Our plan is a lifestyle of changes, remember a la carte. You choose the components that you can start with and use the HyMEP as a map on the journey of QOL. In the Grimoire section (Part 4) are all of the tips to get you started, and the timing, menus and detailed specifics.

The hybrid Mediterranean plan grew out of prepping for the bodybuilding show. I had to come up with some kind of name for this, and as you will see the two doctors Sandy and I have read and whose advice we now follow, Dr. Andrew Weil and Dr. Mehmet Oz, are proponents of just about everything we follow.

There are several different things I would like to list right from the start, but before I do I want to say this eating plan is not that hard, not at all. And you do not have to become a bodybuilder to find the positive results that both Sandy and I have enjoyed.

First though, here are a few key points to know from the beginning. This will be our outline, so to speak, for the HyMEP (Hybrid Mediterranean Eating Plan).

- This eating plan takes some simple effort and planning, and it works!

- It is a long-term, slow-growth change of processes, and change will occur!

- I like to call my lunches and snacks "eating hand food", and saving money!

- Healthy fats that are described in the Grimoire section (Carlson's fish oil and Nutiva Organic coconut oil) are critical—brain health and QOL, baby!

- The mitochondria in our body want good food. They are the power plants of our existence. Insulin resistance is our mortal enemy and kills mitochondria.

- Because sometimes weight gain is related to pre-existing health issues, yes, there might be a medical reason you cannot shave off the weight.

- Favorite foods and how to make your day's worth of food—because it is not lunch!

Sample day's journal from Body Building show, in the Grimoire section, part 4.

Effort and planning

First let me again iterate that I never, did I say NEVER, had any clue or aspiration to train or participate in a bodybuilding show. As things occur in your life, building your educational background, planning for the next phase, remember Indian summer of our adulthood, what the heck are we going to do when we *RETIRE* (I tell you writing that word kind of gives me the heebie-jeebies), ugh, so let's get to it.

I give Sandy all the credit and love in the world for putting up with me during the prep for the show. Not only did she buy all the food, clean all the food, cut up all the veggies and shop at several stores, she had to put up with my borderline OCDness, because as we found out, getting your body fat down to, say three percent, and doing a four-month program can wear on a rela-tionship. For example, I don't know if she will ever allow her husband to do it again because I was such a madman sometimes (no, most of the time).

And that's being nice, really nice.

The first thing that I need everyone to understand, and the first point that we both still adhere to is the timing, that when you eat and how much you eat throughout your day is critical. The show prep is an every-two-hour eating program and I did my best to stick to it; actually in retrospect I did really well. Now that we are in normal mode (thank goodness), small portions happen throughout my day, very regularly, on a three-hour schedule. This is what will keep you on track and more importantly, keep that metabolism cranking.

We all are so conditioned to wait until we are hungry to eat, or the old fashioned three meals a day we were all taught our whole lives, that snacking on trash food, filling up on coffee, grabbing that candy bar or donut, was frankly inevitable!

Let me share the story of how I discovered the Mediterranean diet plan in the first place.

35: Discovering Dr. Weil

While vacationing several years ago, we had, in our vehicle, a book on CD from Dr. Andrew Weil, and so while driving we listened to him—fantastic stuff; I was hooked. When Doctor Weil started to discuss his opinion on this topic I was floored! It was so similar to what we were doing, and we didn't even know it. So, I had to do some investigative reading, and here is what he has to say about this.

From his book *Eating Well for Optimum Health*[25], Dr. Weil talks about the Mediterranean plan as "perhaps the most talked-about diet in recent years", and a "composite of the cuisines of Spain, southern France, Italy, Greece, Crete and parts of the Middle East." Dr. Weil states that "the best-known contemporary of the Mediterranean diet is Walter Willett, Ph.D., chairman of the department of nutrition at the Harvard School of Public Health and co-investigator on the Harvard Nurses study. He is the developer of the Mediterranean Diet Pyramid, which emphasizes olive oil, fish above meat, and cheese above milk.

Mediterranean Diet

Meat &
Sweets

Poultry,
Eggs & Dairy

Seafood

Fruits, Vegetables, Grains,
Olive Oil, Beans, Nuts,
Legumes, Seeds, Herbs & Spices

Key components of the Mediterranean diet

There are also other considerations, according to Dr. Weil, in regard to this type of eating. For example, within the traditional Mediterranean diet there exists a particular cultural context in which people get more physical activity than most Americans. They also enjoy strong social and family bonds around meals—you could say networks or family ties. Eating together and taking pleasure in food are central to these healthy societies. It's not just olive oil. I love the socialization aspect of this eating plan: family, togetherness, talking, sharing stories, and it is something that we all need to make time for. Because it is not only a great way to catch up, relax and enjoy our family time, but the socialization is great for our brain health.

Indeed it is more than olive oil, and the similarities between the HyMEP and the traditional are striking. One of the similarities, and paradoxically speaking, differences is our use of coconut oil as a key healthy fat. Later I will discuss in detail the benefits of coconut oil; however, be aware of the importance of healthy fats, as they are directly related to our energy levels, cell membrane pliability and mitochondria.

Mitochondria: The spark plugs within our body

Mitochondria are the fundamental drivers of metabolism; yes, it is these tiny little cells that power the energy plant.

If someone were to ask you where you get all of your energy, would you answer, "The Snickers bar I just hammered"? Or, "The Mocha Café Grande Cappuccino with whipped cream I just spent six dollars on"? If you did, you are incorrect.

It is our mitochondria.

Mitochondria (we have hundreds per cell) are the conversion machines that take nutrients from the food that we eat and convert them into substances that we need to function, to have energy. You could say they are really important, and they are.

The problem with this arrangement is the function and dysfunction as it relates to aging. Now, suffice to say that you could write entire sections on this phenomenon. Nutrition books are filled with the science behind energy conversion (and if you want a really good read, and much more detail, Google Chris Johnson's *Nutrition* book). However, for our conversation let's keep it brief, and stick to the key facts and my opinion, and how it relates to our dilemma, Boomers.

Mitochondria, when they do their jobs (convert food into useable energy), produce oxygen free radicals—molecules that can cause dangerous inflammation in themselves and the rest of the cells (think back to our conversation and interview with Dr. Lori Shemek on inflammation). Inflammation is a key component of aging, the "rusting" of our pipes (blood vessels) in our cardiovascular system. Is there something we can do to help our mitochondria deal with the ravages of time, and keep them healthy to diffuse the onset of free radicals? The answer, according to a 2003 study by Mayo Clinic researcher Devin Short, Ph.D., is "Yes." Exercise was shown to have a major impact on mitochondrial function. Dr. Short put 65 healthy non-exercisers on a bicycle workout program three days a week. Not only did the participants' aerobic volume increase meaningfully, their mitochondria were generating more ATP-boosting enzymes. (ATP contains high-energy phosphate bonds and is used to transport energy to cells for biochemical processes, including muscle contraction and enzymatic metabolism.)

The efficiency of our mitochondria are critically important to our health; not only are more free radicals produced by inefficient conversion machines (mitochondria), but if this process continues, you continue to not produce energy as efficiently as possible (and a Snickers bar is not going to fix this energy issue). Think of it this way: if our mitochondria can't convert our food into what we need, adenosine triphosphate ATP (energy), we become lethargic, tired, and slow down, and the whole body suffers—not good!

Mitochondria are tiny, but their effects are huge!

Mitochondrial inefficiency has also been linked to brain disease and diabetes, which affects (here we go with the cascading effect of other issues) your pancreas's ability to produce insulin. Some studies have even linked this mitochondrial inefficiency to certain types of Cancer, due to oxidative damage causing DNA damage, and then (as I just said), bam—the big C!

Healthy fat will enable the cell structure to allow the nutrients through the cell wall. Pliability is the key, which then continues the process of mitochondrial conversion of food into our needed ATP.

Understand this one concept, because it has been reported and documented that as we age the efficiency of our mitochondria start to slow, and people over the age of 60 have 40% lower mitochondrial efficiency. The hope is that we will understand the benefits of doing what it takes to keep our tiny power plants humming along. Remember this and possibly improve your longevity and QOL: efficient mitochondria can lead to abundant energy, improved memory, reduced heart disease and potentially – the prevention of cancer. In summary, getting older doesn't have to be all bad.

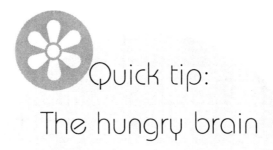

Quick tip: The hungry brain

Starving yourself to lose weight never works. According to researchers at the Albert Einstein College of Medicine, when mice are starved, hunger-sensing neurons break down bits of fat in their own cells to generate energy. This in turn can boost hunger signals.

Night time eating is a sabotage waiting to happen

Understand you are not alone; I battle with this urge at night on a regular basis. Make good decisions. If you must have something to snack on, try this: Greek yogurt with raisins or cottage cheese with cinnamon and Stevia, or I sometimes use fitness bread (Mestemacher) with honey and natural peanut butter. Just don't think you have to feel full; that will take twenty minutes or so, so take the small portion and be patient. Green tea helps take the edge off; a cup at 8:30 or 9:00 really saves me sometimes. Another good option is air-popped popcorn, with coconut oil and sea salt.

Make every carbohydrate meaningful

The 2010 USDA guidelines state 45-65% of carbohydrates are needed, so choose wisely. By that I mean consume complex carbs that contain more fiber than starch, like veggies. Why? Because fiber does not raise your blood sugar and helps you feel satiated (full). Starchy foods (a lot of times they are white in color, a dead giveaway for taboo) do exactly the opposite. Foods that contain starch, like pasta, bread and rice, can send your blood sugar rocketing up. That is a problem, in that rapidly increasing blood sugar triggers our pancreas to jump into action; it is our bodies' sugar regulator, and it sends the insulin army into action. Insulin is a hormone that can trigger the signaling in your body to store fat. It is a Neanderthal brain action—we are hardwired to store in case of famine, when of course there is none, so we get rounder and rounder.

In addition, it is estimated that in around 33% of our population, insulin tends to overshoot its goal. This is a dysfunction that can send our blood sugar plummeting—think of that hungry feeling right after you have eaten; not only has the leptin not kicked in, but the insulin is tricking us into feeling hungry, even though we just had that toast with organic jam.

If you choose your carbohydrates carefully, by eating a better ratio of fiber to calorie and a higher quality of carb, you normalize insulin levels and reduce hunger. A win-win—you eat fewer calories and feel fuller longer. Here are some examples of foods to choose, which fit our HyMEP model: broccoli, Brussels sprouts and peppers are good examples of high-fiber and low-starch (glycemic) foods. Minimally processed foods work well, such as whole fruits rather than canned, whole nuts rather than roasted, whole grains (steel cut oats, barley, quinoa, brown rice) better than processed wheat flour (breakfast cereals).

Making carbohydrates meaningful is the first step in our plan and promotes optimal health. By understanding and developing your plan you are on your way to making better-informed decisions, leaving the autopilot of mindless carbohydrate consumption in the dust.

Lower glycemic (sugar) carbohydrates will lead to lower triglycerides (fat in our blood stream), which can lower our chance at becoming a heart disease case or diabetic.

Eating cleaner

This is becoming a major topic of conversation; the HyMEP will put you in a much better place for achieving a clean diet, and so what is "Clean" exactly?

What we mean when we say clean is this: foods that are produced naturally and are free from processing or synthetic components. Clean foods are free of:

1. Trans-fats

2. Added sweeteners, artificial flavoring, coloring and preservatives

3. Pesticides, herbicides, and pollutants

Since chemicals may affect our health, and we are not sure how they affect our metabolism—and our weight—it is a good idea to avoid these items if possible. That is why it is a good idea to limit processed foods and the buried-in-the-label chemistry. So what are the identifiers of chemistry?

If it comes in a bag, box or is vacuum-sealed or shrink-wrapped, be leery. This is not to say that no good food comes in a package, but be aware are read the label.

If it is made of flour (cereal, bread, crackers, cookies, etc.)

It is a game of learning and it takes a little bit of time; however, think of this: the time you spend reading a label is directly proportional to your QOL and longevity. I like to think of it as the HyMEP longevity factor.

Consuming "good fat"

Hydrogenated oil, or as we refer to them—"trans-fats", have been around a long time.

They were invented in 1897 by Paul Sabatier and refined throughout the early 20th century until "Crisco" was invented in 1914. Trans-fats have no benefit to humans other than as a preservative for food and a longer shelf life for items like crackers and cookies. These are used in many products; read labels, because they are buried in processed foods. Trans-fats have been linked to a range of health conditions including higher LDL cholesterol levels and obesity.

Saturated fats have been given a bad rap in the past; marketing and the dreaded diets that are seemingly invented daily will sometimes lead you to believe that eating fat is bad for you, but this is not true. One of the worst and most insidious food labels ever to be invented is the "fat-free" moniker. It painted the picture of over-indulgence as long as it was "fat-free", that quality and quantity of calories and sugar do not matter, and that is completely untrue. Without the natural filling quantities of calories from fat in foods, the stripped down "fat-free" substitutes left you hungrier and forced you to consume chemicals and additives (sugar, salt, and thickeners) to make the food taste good.

Natural fat is good for your body; even animal fat, in balanced quantities, can be good for you. You can choose many different types of natural fats, and incorporating them into your diet and can be hugely beneficial. You need anywhere from 20-35% of your daily calories from quality fat. Later in the book you will read more on how I incorporate specific fat consumption, and how the bodybuilding show's "slow-glide prep" proved to me how to get the most out of my calories, but for now think of these:

- Coconut and olive oil

- Free-range meats, like beef, poultry and pork, raised on their natural foods, not corn or soy products

- Fatty fruits, for example avocado and olives

- Nuts and seeds

- Fish

A University of Connecticut study found that eating these foods while cutting bad carbs reduces key factors for heart disease, and does so more effectively than a low-fat diet.

Cheat days—Make them work for you!

One of the first health books I ever read was Bill Phillips' *Body for Life*[26] book; I like to think he motivated a huge number of people to turn the corner as far as fitness and nutrition. His concept of a one-day cheat session works, and here is why: No one wants to go through life deprived; it sets us up for bingeing and creates havoc for our intention of living a healthy and balanced lifestyle. Cheat days, if you stick to them, can be a reward day for a strong week. I like to use Sunday as my cheat day; it removes that anxiety and feeling of sacrifice. You should live a meaningful and happy life, and diets that restrict your total calories and do not address the human side of reward will fail. Just remember balance; balance is the key—you earn it, so let it work for you, not against you. Responsibility, common sense and personal account-ability, along with our HyMEP will work, but it is not a quick fix; it is a lifestyle change that will give you the map to a long and healthy life.

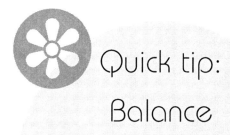

Quick tip:

Balance

Of all the changes taking place on the food and nutrition front, one of the most important issues is the balance between diet and body movement (exercise).

Ben Goldacre wrote in his book Bad Science[27] that "We have somehow become collectively obsessed with these absurd, thinly evidenced individuals' tinkerings in diet, distracting us from simple, healthy eating ad-vice but, more than that, as we saw, distracting us from the other important lifestyle risk factors for ill health that cannot be sold or commodified."

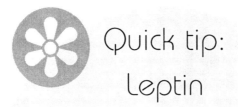

Quick tip: Leptin

Leptin is your bodies' long-term regulator, which is produced in fat cells; it tells
the brain that the bodies' fat reserves are
sufficient by signaling the hypothalamus
and quieting appetite signals. The issue
lies in the fact that although obese people have plenty of Leptin, they just do not
respond to its signals correctly.

More on the Mediterranean Diet

The Mediterranean diet lowers our mortality rate by
25%, and along with exercise, by 28%.

The Mediterranean diet emphasizes:

- Getting plenty of exercise

- Eating primarily plant-based foods, such as
  fruits and vegetables, whole grains, legumes and
  nuts

- Replacing butter with healthy fats such as olive
  oil and canola oil

- Using herbs and spices instead of salt to flavor
  foods

- Limiting red meat to no more than a few times a month

- Eating fish and poultry at least twice a week

- Drinking red wine in moderation (optional)

- The diet also recognizes the importance of enjoying meals with family and friends.

http://www.mayoclinic.com/health/Mediterranean-diet/CL00011

The Do-Nots of the HyMEP:

As I made better and newer choices, and became much more informed as far as my food consumption and the way I felt, I saw the results in improvements of my key numbers, for example cholesterol and blood pressure. I realized that certain regulars in my eating habits had drastically changed. I had eliminated and/or substituted several regular items, and I want to share those with you, for example:

- Soda: diet and regular

First I want to be up front and completely honest, as I have done throughout this book. I liked–no, let me emphasize LOVED—Coke Zero. I thought its predecessor Diet Coke was the ultimate, until the new and improved version showed up. It was love at first drink, and that is the problem—it's really good. Too bad it is so bad for me! Now I wanted to keep this section on my "NO LONGER IN MY EATING AND DRINKING" concise, so I am not going into all of the science of each of these items, just understand I no longer drink soda, at all.

- Alcoholic beverages

As I have openly shared, and always will, I am a problem drinker. So the no alcohol is a no-brainer for me. For you, understand that for any results in improvement of your nutrition, empty calories—for example alcoholic beverages—are out. Give yourself a 30-day trial with this, and watch what happens. Substitute water, tea, or mineral water and give yourself a shot at losing some pounds; you may be really surprised at the outcome.

- If it is white, it is probably not right!

White food has been almost completely dropped from my eating. With the exception of air-popped popcorn, we have mostly eliminated white foods like bread, sugar (remember inflammation), and table salt (we now use sea salt).

I have inadvertently become somewhat gluten-free. Not that I was trying, however, there is a lot of information on gluten intolerance in our eating, and much information on this topic everywhere you look.

- Fast Food

Our love affair with fast food is crushing us, and I mean both by weight and financially. The attitude of "I don't have time" is our own making—hate to say it. Fast food should be eaten sparingly if at all, and children and their burgeoning obesity issue should be a huge red flag to all of us. Eating in a car was a novelty when we were young; now it has evolved into a creature that threatens all of us through becoming hooked on salt and fat. Become accountable and limit your Big Mac attack, and super sizing something is only making us all super-sized people. Fast food is by far the easiest, most convenient, and most common way for the average person to eat too many calories. Where else can you get a 2000 calorie meal for under $15 without even getting out of your car?

Despite the many gimmicks, fad diets and seemingly infinite sources of bad information, the single biggest factor in weight control is calories. More specifically, the relationship between how many calories your body burns per day and how many calories you consume (as in eat or drink) per day. What I mean is...

- Consuming more calories than you burn = weight gain

- Burning more calories than you consume = weight loss

- Consuming and burning the same number of calories = weight maintenance

So, if you currently have weight to lose or just want to prevent yourself from ever having weight to lose, the most important and all around useful thing you can do diet-wise is pay attention to your calorie intake.

The thing is, one of the most common food choices for the average person is fast food. That's a fact. And, as if this is going to be a shock to anyone on the planet, fast food is one of the worst high-calorie offenders. That's another fact. The combination of these two facts is... well... not so good.

Now, while I can't stop fast food eateries from selling foods that are pathetically high in calories, and I certainly can't stop people from eating fast food (it's convenient, cheap and tasty, I know), what I can attempt to do is help in the making of better choices. Or, in this case, prevent the making of the worst ones.

Full disclosure

I loved McDonalds; my favorite meal was a Quarter Pounder with Cheese, 510 calories, Filet-o-Fish sandwich, 380 calories, Super-size large fries, 540 calories, and a large chocolate shake, 505 calories, with a total of 1935 calories. In addition, Wendy's, Kentucky Fried Chicken, Burger King and probably every other fast food outlet saw me at one time or another. Oh, and did I mention eating late at night after going to the bars way back in the dark ages? I think we all have had our moments; the chemistry of fast food is tasty, the results are not.

The FAQ

How many calories should we eat per day?

This question is dependent upon your age, size and activity level, and here are some good tips to get you rolling. I have used these tips myself and these really do work; it is amazing how just the smallest of snacks add up and just pulverize our efforts.

- First, keep a food journal for three days—everything! At this point you can use a calorie calculator like an app called "Lose it" or try fitday.com. This will give us our starting number; we have got to have this data, so be honest and write down everything you put in your mouth. Now we have a starting number, good. This is hard but we have got to know this.

- Next is our amount of calories we actually need based on our activity level

If you do not work out at all, multiply your body weight by 10; so for example a 150-pound person would need 1500 calories.

- If you work out twice a week, then adjust the number to 12; so now your calorie count is 1800.

- If you work out three or four times a week, adjust the number to 14; so now you are at 2100.

- If you work out five or more times, a week adjust to 16; so now we are at 2400.

So, now you have raw numbers. Data is always important, and for lifestyle changes, a must. A 170-calorie deficit per day, whatever your daily total is, will equate to a one-pound loss a week—as you can see, it really is pretty straightforward. So now we have a simple system; deficit is a way to improvement, so find the "holes" in your day. By that I mean those times when we can gain a small number toward the objective, eliminate unnecessary snacks, and by timing your day correctly you should not need the Snickers bar.

Processed foods

If it comes from a box, or a bag, and has more ingredients than a child's chemistry set you may want to slow your pace down on eating or drinking these products. Notice I said "slow down"; the HyMEP is all about behavior modification, not quick fixes.

Processed foods (which SOME in my opinion have small amounts of nutritional value) are so prevalent and so inexpensive and taste so good that it would be difficult to just drop them from our lives—let's be real here. Let's crawl before we walk, and walk before we run; this type of change is, again, a slow process. We did not put on 30 or 40 pounds overnight; the HyMEP is NOT a quick fix, but it will work.

Remember HyMEP is an eating plan, not a diet!

I want to add a thought toward our food industry, or the industrialization of our food. The food giants, for example General Mills, are in the business of food, and I believe that when it comes right down to it they make a variety of products to support a variety of needs, economically and financially.

They have taken what is our governments' policy toward agriculture and crop production and maximized their return on investment. If a box of cereal has four cents worth of raw material (corn) and they can sell it for four dollars, then good for them. They do make great products, along with the not so nutritionally great. Understand this though: *and this is the major point here;* no one forces you to buy it and then eat it!

That is an individual choice, period!

Accountability needs to be understood and addressed. Quit blaming the food giants; if people don't buy their products, the economic laws will create a change.

Eating Lucky Charms did not make you fat. Eating Lucky Charms every day for a year did.

Medical—and Health-related weight issues

I do want to give my thoughts on a few medical reasons that you may be experiencing a tough time with your weight, if all of the dieting and exercise just is not getting it done. There potentially could be a medical reason for this and you should consult your physician.

For example;

- Thyroid issues

- Food allergies

- Pre- or post-menopausal issues

- Hormonal issues, including low testosterone

If you have been experiencing a weight gain, or have a really tough time losing any weight at all it may not be as simple as the law of thermodynamics and calories in and out. It is very possible that you may have one of the above conditions. I encourage anyone who is suffering with a weight issue, who is doing their best due diligence as far as movement and eating correctly, to seek assistance from their physician. Your numbers and blood work can shed light on a condition that may be deeper than just burning more calories than you consume. Don't procrastinate—we all need to encourage all of our boomer brothers and sisters to be as happy as possible, and to live that QOL we talk about so much. Get your physical.

36: Did Captain Crunch sink our ship?

I had this thought one day about what we did as kids that really got us into this obesity issue in the first place. I mean, all of this eating and overweight-ness had to start somewhere, right? Understanding where a problem started helps us in the process of education and improvement. I mean, really, did we all become addicted to sugar by drinking breast milk or baby formula?

I wrote a blog called "Did Captain Crunch Sink our Ship?", and really it was an idea about our love affair with sugar, that stat of how much sugar we (on average) consume now compared to say, 300 years ago, is something like this[28]:

1700 AD	4 lbs
1800 AD	18 lbs
1900 AD	90 lbs
2000 AD	145 lbs (yikes)

And according to Michael Polin, author of a fabulous book, *The Omnivore's Dilemma*[29], our sugar consumption number, including all sugars (which includes sugar from cane, beet, glucose, honey, maple syrup and the like, although high-fructose corn syrup is the leader of the pack), has gone from 128 pounds per person in 1985 to 158 pounds today.

Double yikes!

Significant, outrageous, or how about plain old ridiculous? It's no wonder we have an obesity problem, which leads to a diabetes problem, which leads to a cardiovascular problem, which leads to a coronary problem, which leads to a brain problem, which leads to a death problem.

It's a problem!

The Food Pyramid

If Captain Crunch didn't sink our ships then it may have been a torpedo from—of all places—the USDA. Yes, the United States Department of Agriculture. Research has shown that the food pyramid, developed by the U.S. Department of Agriculture in 1992, advises daily consumption of six to 11 servings of bread, cereal, rice, and pasta; two to three servings of meat, poultry, fish, dry beans, eggs, and nuts; and sparing consumption of fats, oils, and sweets. Balanced and looking out for all of us, the food pyramid is a disaster, and the torpedo that has set us up for an obesity epidemic.

The food pyramid was published widely across the United States. It's printed on cereal boxes and bread wrappers, posted on elementary school bulletin boards, and published in university textbooks. It's also known globally. The USA Rice Federation distributes the food pyramid, for example, through its promotion of U.S. rice in Mexico. But the food pyramid is outdated and doesn't reflect the latest food research; that is according to research done by Dr. Walter Willett, (mentioned earlier with Dr. Weil) a leading U.S. nutrition researcher, in his book *Eat, Drink and Be Healthy: The Harvard Medical School Guide to Healthy Eating*[30]. Dr. Willett states that the "food pyramid, considered almost holy by many nutritionists and dieters, is wrong and hurts both waistlines and health," and that "the USDA food pyramid serves the interests of its main client, the U.S. agricultural industry"!

If you read *The Omnivore's Dilemma (IBID 29)* or *Fast Food Nation*[31] you will see that other researchers agree with Dr. Willett that USDA has been buffaloed into believing big food lobbying. According to Dr. Willet, "At best, the USDA Pyramid offers indecisive, scientifically unfounded advice on an absolutely vital topic--what to eat. At worst, the misinformation it offers contributes to overweight, poor health, and unnecessary early deaths."

USA Today reported that a startling 61% of U.S. citizens weigh too much, and about 26% are obese -30 pounds or more over a healthy weight. Willett says that the USDA pyramid puts too much emphasis on red meat and lumps too many types of carbohydrates together. The pyramid gives too little emphasis to nuts, beans, and healthy oils, which have positive health effects. Willett's alternative, the Healthy Eating Pyramid, emphasizes eating plant oils like olive, canola, and soy, and suggests eating lots of vegetables while giving fish, poultry, and eggs a higher profile than red meat.

It's interesting how similar his program is to our HyMEP, with the emphasis on healthy fats, hand food veggies which are complex carbohydrates, simple carbs like fruit and limiting red meat matching our lifestyle program. That and moving more can add up to a much healthier society. It really does come full circle to what we already know. Follow what our grandmothers told us and you will be healthier; it is not rocket science—it is very straight forward[32].

The scoop on poop

I am the kind of dad that is really into poop; I am going to admit that right here and now. Before you get all repulsed and grossed out, listen to this story—and as always, it's all true. From Captain Crunch to the Food Pyramid the next result is of course, yes you guessed it, poop.

When my oldest daughter Ashley was born (a blessing), I was a typical first-time clueless parent. Birthing classes that were the rage in the mid-'80s were in full swing, and yes I did my duty and attended. (My question now, some 25 years later is, are they still as boring?) I wanted to be a great dad. She was perfectly healthy, even a tad large at over nine pounds.

Getting that child home was non cinch, I mean car seats and all; did I say I was clueless?

Anyway, for the first three months that we had this infant it was tough. She cried, a lot, and especially at night, and lucky me because I worked nights at that time, I got to care for the li'l bundle of pain in the assness. Have you ever been around a kid who cried all night long? I had to walk her every single night until she fell asleep. I knew something was not right, but being the clueless dad that I was...

Have you ever heard of colic? Neither had I, and this is where I became a reader of poop, but first the medical definition:

The strict medical definition of colic is a condition of a healthy baby in which it shows periods of intense, unexplained fussing/crying lasting more than 3 hours a day, more than 3 days a week for more than 3 weeks![33]

This is serious stuff, I mean marriages can suffer, babies suffer, injuries occur; I have to emphasize how bad this really sucks! It was terrible.

So when the doctor explained to me that looking at the poop, and understanding the physical characteristics of the child's excrement (in know-nothing parental terms, turds), yellow cottage cheese-looking stuff is not what we want—that is not what a turd should look like; it is a pain in the ass and your babies tummy, and in essence, "Colic".

I became an expert on the science of children's "poop". Which of course leads us to becoming an expert of 'Poopology', and my fascination with admiring your daily duty, and my sharing this valuable information with you.

Admire your work.

"Don't be so trigger-happy with the flusher. Turn around and take a look at your poop, which speaks volumes about your gut and overall health. Poop should be smooth and S-shaped, like your colon. If it comes out lumpy, or drops into the bowl like marbles, you're constipated; increase your fiber and water intake."

~Dr. Mehmet Oz

I don't want to frighten anyone, but here are some facts on being irregular. And being that this whole book is on quality of life, and I am fastidious as it pertains to poop, we all need to know more about this, even though my children think I am a complete freak!

Effects of Chronic Irregularity

This fact shocks most people. This is because so many people walk around constipated they don't realize what being regular means. There are many consequences of not being regular. Irregularity can have devastating effects on the body and the colon. Here are just a few effects of irregularity:

Hemorrhoids, or worse, anal fissures (anal what?), which can cause pain and rectal bleeding both externally and internally. Most people who develop these conditions actually experience more constipation because it becomes painful to have a bowel movement, so they avoid one.

Impacted feces (Ugh!), a condition where feces become so hardened it becomes stuck in the bowel, forming an obstruction. This can be dangerous, and can result in bacteria growing within the bowels in some cases. In other cases it can cause a person to strain so hard they develop a hernia.

Development of cancers of the colon (this is getting ridiculous), which may result from long-term impacted fecal matter.

Clogged lymph nodes, poor skin, and ill-functioning kidneys (compounding issues), all resulting from the lack of ability to remove waste matter from the body. Decreased energy and lethargy.

Chronic pain or malaise (I could say "no shit" here, but I won't), including joint pain or muscle pain. Some people develop arthritis-like conditions.

Problems with the gallbladder.

No wonder there are so many laxative commercials, dang!

Regular versus irregular, why are all the ads on the nightly news dominated by irregularity? If your daily duty is daily, if the regularity is regular, if you are not bound by that bound-up feeling, then good for you, keep it going, and keep it flushing.

There really is nothing funny about being bound up and hurting!

In Conclusion

I have tried to keep this as concise and somewhat short as possible; however, please understand that as far as nutrition and weight management is concerned I have been there and done that.

Cutting down on bad fat, and even worse, bad carbs (Captain Crunch did not do us any favors), is going to give you some better odds in the long run, and that is what we are aiming for. A diet low in bad saturated fat and the refined sugars may reduce our risk of developing dementia, according to many studies. Some studies have shown that people tested who had been on a low-glycemic, low-fat food regimen performed better on memory tests, and calorie-restrictive diets are getting some serious looks. Other studies have shown that the Mediterranean diet, similar to our hybrid, which is high in good saturated fats, nuts, fish, coconut and olive oils, fruits and vegetables could cut our Alzheimer's risk. I cover more in-depth analysis on Alzheimer's later, but suffice to say that as we age and live longer it is going to be as Dr. Bartzokis taught me, better odds, better odds!

I have shared all of the routes, paths, clues and mistakes I have had to endure. As I said toward the end of the Captain Crunch section I would love to hear success stories and your input, and help share the knowledge. Tell us what worked for you, because, my friends, it is all about sharing and helping each other.

My sample days are very doable. Remember, in our Grimoire section 4 is the complete list, but here are the golden rules

- Small steps to success

- There is no quick fix

- The HyMEP, Hybrid-Mediterranean Eating Plan, works!

- Water, water, water

- Balance is key; limited amounts of processed foods can be okay in a balanced eating plan

Being fifty pounds overweight is no fun (I know that from personal experience), and more than that must be very tough; my heart goes out to you. I want to assist you in losing that weight and improving your QOL; it is the whole reason for writing this book!

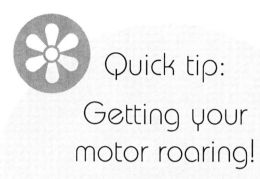

Quick tip:

Getting your motor roaring!

Eat frequent, small meals. Long periods between meals signal that your body should retain calories—in the form of fat—to sustain life when food isn't available. By eating frequently, you let your body know everything is okay and it should just burn the food rather than storing it.[34]

37: Graduate school

As I finished my undergraduate work at Michigan State in 2006, at the ripe young age of 46, I had actually been contemplating this grad-school thing. Even though the beginning of going back to school in the first place had been such a daunting experience, I felt good about how I finished. That is a point I want to hammer home right now, Boomers. When you do, it is challenging, maybe even overwhelming. Don't let it scare you off. Being at our stage of life, we have the mental capacity to overcome. I mean, come on, we have lived a lot longer than the traditional students, and let me tell you a secret—they are more afraid of us than we are of them. Reach out and become part of the proverbial student tribe.

Your skillset will come back, and actually improve, because you appreciate the opportunity a hell of a lot more than when you were younger, and, frankly, less experienced (I was going to say dumber, but that would be negative.); I know I certainly did. Again, it is through mentors and advice that the whole process takes place; I sought out advice from people I admired and trusted, and they gave me really good counsel. Seek out help. I was a little bit afraid, but so what?

It is all about prep work; just like anything else, planning is the key. So I visited people who knew the system, figured it out and started prepping. First thing – affirmations; tell people your goal, write it down and then attack. They have this thing called the GRE; it is an exam that is administered for many graduate programs, a nationally recognized exam, and frankly a bitch. I am not going to say it was anything it was not, and I don't want to discourage anyone from attempting this. Remember, if I can pass this thing... anyone can; it was all in the prep work, and this is where we boomers excel, with desire and planning. So I looked at the summer before I took this thing as a summer school class, no different than what I had just finished, using time management, studying x number of hours a day and a week, figuring out the plan and then BOOM—implementation.

Okay, so you start, and get going with this, another mountain, another goal. This time, however, the stakes are higher; there is a deadline, and there is either a thesis or a comprehensive exam to finish, so this is reallllllly the big leagues. Things are completely different though; you have a full Professor as an advisor—mine was Johannes Bauer, and he is an intimidating cat to say the least. To be perfectly honest, at first I was intimidated by his intellect and no-nonsense approach;

the guy is an off-the-charts global genius, exactly what I needed; however, at that moment, I did not have a clue. I have been blessed to have tough coaches who pushed really hard, he knew I had it, and they pushed the right buttons. I think that's why I am such a good coach now, having been coached up by some studs, anyway.

I had a three-year deadline; even though you have five to complete this coursework, I told my other key mentor, Dr. Roy Simon that I would complete this in three years. He answered that many others had sought his advice and not followed through, and so I had to have a deadline. Set one for yourself; it works. I had it all figured out, had a thesis idea, and I was going to change the world – wrong, Whippersnapper. Professor Bauer read my proposal, and he read the re-writes, the re-written re-writes, and said, "Sorry, Son; not good enough, too broad." So being that I was 46, as any good advisor will do, he convinced me to get on with the coursework and take the comprehensive, which meant an extra 10 course work credits and then the mind numbing comp, ugh! Another exam, damn; no get around these guys—did I say big leagues?

I figured I had to earn Professor Bauer's respect, so I took his classes, and let me tell you this guy does not mess around. However, in grad school, something funny happened. I realized I could do this. I mean, confidence is one half the battle, so if it takes grinding and office hours, so be it. I visited my professors more than any traditional student ever did! They were going to know me, my family, my work ethic, my plight, everything. Remember, I mentioned this earlier, office hours are the greatest; use them—they are there for a reason and traditional students... well, they don't seem to understand how much you can learn from these men and women.

Classes, all of them were insanely hard, but none like my very last course. I mean, if you recall earlier I had talked about the illness that started this whole life-changing epiphany, remember? That was my second year of grad school, spring 2008. I had two courses and still four-pointed them both, even after missing two weeks of class (being on top of your game will come in handy when the grim reaper comes calling).

My final course, which I thought would help me in the comp exam, was a media economics course, taught by Professor Steve Wildman, a Stanford educated 'badass'. His intellect was on the same level as Professor Bauer; I mean, these guys are so 'fricking' smart it is utterly ridiculous, in any event. I had the one course and study time for this comp thing, so it was a very trying spring of 2009. It turns out that Professor Wildman's course was just not jiving with me; his economics problems were crazy hard for me, and I just had a really tough time with it. Again, two things saved my ass: office hours (we got to be really good friends because I bothered him so much) and the project, a paper that I could actually wrap my head around. There was a point halfway through the semester when I thought I was going to fail the course—the mid-term. I tanked it—just froze and tanked... no other excuse.

Well, somehow, through the grace of the higher being, I made it through both the class and the exam, and graduated. It was exhilarating to say the least; this was something I never, ever thought about trying, and now my children saw their dad walk and wear the black robe. And even better than that, it was a non-planned double graduation because Ashley, my oldest daughter, finished her bachelor's the same semester. So dad and daughter graduated the same weekend from the same University; it could not have been any sweeter.

The moral to this is—when you think you cannot move forward with a goal, think of me—just a regular guy who had a chance and made the most of it. It has led to many bigger and better things.

Part 3:

ACTIVITY (30%)

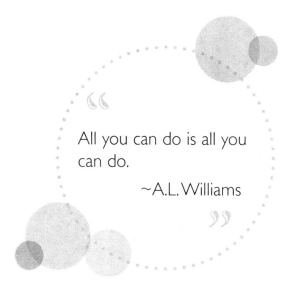

> " All you can do is all you can do.
>
> ~A.L. Williams "

This country is primed for a health revolution, with Boomers leading the way. At seventy-nine million strong, work ethic and longevity, experience, wisdom and now reaching the pinnacle of their lives, this point in our world history is primed for the next revolution.

While some factors, such as your genes, are out of your control, many powerful lifestyle factors are within your sphere of influence. Healthy tips to think about:

The six pillars of a brain-healthy lifestyle are:

1. Regular exercise

2. A healthy diet

3. Mental stimulation

4. Quality sleep

5. Stress management

6. An active social life

When it comes to our lives and the quality we so richly deserve, one of the major issues I have continually discussed on the talk show is brain health, specifically dementia and Alzheimer's. Movement, staying busy, social awareness, connectedness, sleep and managing stress are of paramount importance to managing these debilitating conditions. I believe this is so important that starting this section with these topics is tops on my list. In my interviews with all of my neuroscience and psychologist family members, movement is the top item in battling age-related diseases.

I have had the pleasure to interview Dr. P. Murali Doraiswamy twice on "Boomers Rock", and his expertise and input is invaluable. He, along with Dr. George Bartzokis (mentioned several times earlier), make a formidable team of intellect and have helped increase my knowledge and importance of sharing the message of giving yourself those "better odds" as we all move into our perpetual Indian summer of our lives. Because dementia and Alzheimer's are age-related conditions, we as a population, boomers specifically, need to become acutely aware of this impending time bomb.

Dr. Murali Doraiswamy, M.D., is a renowned expert on brain health and an expert on brain aging and mental health. He is the head of Duke University's biological psychiatry division and a Senior Fellow at Duke University's Center for the Study of Aging. As director of psychiatry clinical trials at Duke for nearly 10 years, he received numerous awards for his work as an investigator on landmark studies. The author of more than 200 scientific articles, Dr. Doraiswamy has served as an advisor to the Food and Drug Administration, the American Federation for Aging Research, the National Institute on Aging, and the World Health Organization, as well as leading Alzheimer's medical journals and advocacy groups. His research has been featured in the *Wall Street Journal, USA Today,* and the *New York Times,* and on *CBS News,* the *Today Show, NPR and the BBC.*

As Dr. D. stated in his book, *The Alzheimer's Action Plan*[35]:

Dementia is the broad general diagnosis given to a person whose thinking, particularly memory, is so impaired it affects day-to-day functioning. Not all dementia is due to Alzheimer's, but everyone with Alzheimer's has dementia. However, the term 'Alzheimer's' is often used incorrectly to refer to different types of dementia that impair memory and occur in older individuals. More than a hundred different disorders cause dementia, and their different symptoms depend on what parts of the brain they attack. Many Alzheimer's experts tell and advise patients that what is good for the heart-healthy weight, daily exercise, no smoking, a good diet (which includes plenty of whole foods, fruits and vegetables), and a social network, is good for your brain.

Will it, in fact, help us boomers? That, my friends, is the 65 million dollar question!

Shrinking Hippocampus, Memory Loss, and Alzheimer's—Study

Using magnetic resonance imaging, Mayo Clinic researchers found that specific changes in the hippocampus were linked to changes in behavior associated with aging and Alzheimer's disease. "When certain parts of the hippocampus shrink or deteriorate, specific, related memory abilities are affected," says neurologist Ronald C. Petersen[36], the principal author of the study. Dr. John Ratey calls the hippocampus the cartographer of our brain, the super librarian; it is the memory indexer, so a shrunken brain librarian/director and consolidator of new memories (hippocampus) is a stepping stone to the great unknown, literally[37].

In addition, individuals with a shrunken hippocampus tend to progress more rapidly toward Alzheimer's. "In earlier studies we were able to show that the volume of the hippocampus could help diagnose early Alzheimer's disease or help predict which patients may develop Alzheimer's disease in the future. Now we can look specifically at which (part or parts) of the hippocampus are affected and match that with particular memory functions which are impaired in that particular patient," says Dr. Petersen. As the number of Alzheimer's cases in the U.S. continues to rise, urgency is setting in. Who wants to live to a hundred if you can't remember your name, your address or how to drive your car? The Alzheimer's diagnosis is now shared by 5.4 million Americans, and that stat is sure to rise; some estimates put it at 100 million, globally, by 2050.

The Alzheimer's Association calls the illness "the defining disease of baby boomers"!

For us it is critical to know whether lifestyle changes will make a difference, and the answer is difficult to pin down.

In a white paper Dr. Doriaswamy forwarded to me before our interview on "Boomers Rock", the link between fitness and Alzheimer's was clearly proposed. The title "Fitness and the Brain: Can a Walk a Day Keep Alzheimer's Away", was enlightening, to say the least. Dr. Doriaswamy's article, dated November 2008, stated how scientists are excited about the prospects of physical activity and movement as a "strategy" for lowering risk factors for dementia such as blood pressure, cholesterol, diabetes and depression. Some studies are supplying evidence that movement and light exercise can be beneficial. One such study published in 2008 by Nicola Lautenschlager and colleagues from the University of Western Australia[38] sought to validate this way of thinking.

Here is what they discovered.

With 170 older people in this study (a small effect size; however, interesting data was gleaned), with memory complaints of 60% cognitive loss, severe enough to be diagnosed with mild cognitive impairment, these people were put into the program study and here is the resulting quote from Dr. Doriaswamy's article:

"Over the next six months, half of the study participants were assigned to a home-based exercise program. They were encouraged to do at least three 50-minute sessions of exercise (mostly walking) each week. Those who were already doing this level of exercise at study entry (about 25%) were asked to up their activity level by an additional 50 minutes. The other half were assigned to receive basic health education as a control group. At the end of six months, exercisers improved modestly (scoring about 20% higher than controls) on an overall measure of cognitive abilities. The subgroup of people with mild cognitive impairment also improved. One year after the trial ended, the exercisers still sustained a 10% edge on overall cognitive score compared with controls and also had significantly less decline on a memory measure. A host of other cognitive sub-tests did not differ between the groups, however."

"The study is important because it is the first to demonstrate that exercise benefits cognition in *older* adults with subjective and objective memory problems over 18 months."

Some articles have been written stating that Alzheimer's is the second most feared disease, after cancer. With over five million people living with this (and there is no cure), any and all action is needed to head off this impending disaster.

Scientists know Alzheimer's damages and destroy brain cells; they also know that age, family history and genetics can increase your chances for developing the disease.

Dr. George Bartzokis, the UCLA neurologist and Alzheimer's expert mentioned earlier in the book, asked me in a pre-interview phone call for the radio show how old I hoped to live to? I thought about it and said hopefully to 100. He said, "Okay, so what do you think your odds are of acquiring Alzheimer's?" I thought about this and said, "if you are asking me this it must be pretty high; how about fifty percent!" Dr. George responded, "Try seventy to eighty!"

Alzheimer's is age dependent!

As researchers like Dr. Bartzokis work to raise awareness and funding for continued research, there may be some strategies and steps to reduce our odds and risk.

Here are three:

Exercise- At the Alzheimer's Association International Conference, researchers reported on roughly how many cases of Alzheimer's may be attributable to certain behaviors or conditions; in the USA, physical *inactivity* topped the list. Regular exercise and movement keeps your cardiovascular system healthy, which is good for your heart and your brain. Some studies suggest that regular movement and/or structured exercise may directly benefit brain cells due to the increased oxygen and blood flow.

Control your blood sugar- A study published in the journal *Neurology* showed that people with diabetes are twice as likely to develop Alzheimer's as people with normal blood sugar levels (glucose). That is because high blood sugar and insulin resistance may lead to complications that could harm brain cells directly or damage the blood supply (vessels) that deliver oxygen and nutrients to the brain.

Have your Cholesterol checked- Scientists in Japan discovered that people who have high cholesterol levels were more likely to have markers in the brain that are identified as plaques. This is in comparison to those who have normal or lower cholesterol levels. Another motivation to watch your cholesterol, as damage to your circulatory system and heart from high cholesterol appears to increase your odds of Alzheimer's.

38: Can we afford this?

Building a movement of people who care, enlightened education, and preventive actions may be our best plan of attack in dealing with early-onset dementia and Alzheimer's. By that I mean what we have been talking about earlier—more movement, improvements in our diets, treating and eliminating the early risk factors; we have to understand. I hope that with all of the discussion we had earlier in the book on brain physiology, neurogenesis, plasticity and myelin, along with the behavioral information, that the picture is becoming clearer; this is important information, and I certainly don't want to have to deal with this, and my hope is you will not either. Either for myself or as a caregiver, what to do?

Become more educated and accountable; financially this thing is a freight train rumbling down our track of life. I, for one, do not want to get run over!

This financial freight train could ruin us all.

Dr. Bartzokis and I talked about this in our pre-interview call, the impending costs of all of these "centenarians" (those people who are 100 years old), with potential to develop Alzheimer's and dementia, since it is known that these diseases are reportedly linked to age and longevity. If we think our healthcare system is in trouble now, read on; this is not a pretty picture.

Costs

According to the Alzheimer's Association, the average lifetime cost for an Alzheimer's patient is $174,000. In 2011, the overall cost of health care, long term and hospice was $183 billion; by 2050 that cost is expected to skyrocket to $1.1 trillion.

On average it costs about $21 dollars a day nationally for home health care, adult day care is around $70 dollars a day and a nursing care facility with a private room is close to $90,000 a year (prices vary according to states), which is considered custodial care and NOT covered by Medicare. Long-term care insurance is an option, but as we get older the cost is going to go higher[39].

We need to plan better, understand our options and work together in solving this; we have choices, and I want to maximize mine. We also need to give and help people like Dr. Bartzokis with fundraising and awareness.

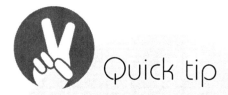 Quick tip

Walk a mile a day. Or bike or swim or try any aerobic exercise that burns calories and strengthens the heart. Heart disease is the nation's leading killer. More than 40 percent of U.S. adults can expect to suffer from cardiovascular disease by 2030, with medical bills exceeding $1 trillion. More than half of those costs will be borne by Medicare. Extra exercise cuts the nation's medical bill.

39: Centenarians

Life expectancy in the United States has continually been on the increase with the advance of medicine and healthier lifestyles. In conjunction with this increase, the number of individuals 100 years old or greater, or centenarians, has also increased.

According to the US Census Bureau:

- In 1990, there were 37,306 centenarians in the United States, or 1 per 6,667 people, roughly 15 per 100,000.

- In 2000, there were 50,454 centenarians in the United States, or 1 per 5,578 people, roughly 18 per 100,000.

The Census Bureau estimates there were 71,991 centenarians as of Dec. 1, 2010, up from 37,306 two decades earlier. While predicting longevity and population growth is difficult, the census' low-end estimate for 2050 is 265,000 centenarians; its highest projection puts the number at 4.2 million.

"They have been the fastest-growing segment of our population in terms of age," said Thomas Perls, director of the New England Centenarian Study at Boston University.

The rising number of centenarians is not just a byproduct of the nation's growing population —they make up a bigger chunk of it. In 1990, about 15 in every 100,000 Americans had reached 100; in 2010, it was more than 23 per 100,000, according to census figures.

Perls said the rise in 100-year-olds is attributed largely to better medical care and the dramatic drop in childhood-mortality rates since the early 1900s. Centenarians also have good genes on their side, he said, and have made common-sense health decisions, such as not smoking and keeping their weight down. Socialization, working, and staying active and engaged all are traits that not only can help us live longer, but better.

As we have firmly entered the 21st century, population aging has emerged as a major demographic trend worldwide. Declining fertility, and improved health and longevity, have swelled the older populations dramatically—and at an unprecedented rate[40].

More stats

Consider:

- For the first time in history, people aged 65 and over will soon outnumber children under the age of 5.

- Throughout the world today, there are more people aged 65 and older than the entire populations of Russia, Japan, France, Germany and Australia—combined.

- By 2030, 55 countries are expected to see their 65 and older populations become at least 20 percent of their total.

- By 2040, the global population is projected to number 1.3 billion older people—accounting for 14 percent of the total.

- By 2050, the U.N. estimates that the proportion of the world's population age 65 and over will more than double, from 7.6% today to 16.2%[41].

- Today in the U.S. there are approximately 40.3 million Americans are age 65 and older, an estimated 13% of the population, according to the U.S. Census Bureau. Their number is expected to more than double to 89 million by 2050.

This bodes a dire situation for the Social Security system and other entitlement programs, which are in a financial quagmire. When Social Security was announced in the Roosevelt administration in 1935 there were 163 people contributing to the fund for every person receiving it. By 1950 that number had dropped to a little more than 15 people contributing to every person receiving benefits, and it is estimated that in the next fifteen years that number shift to two people for every recipient. In 1940 the retirement age was established at 65, and the life expectancy was on average 62.9, now the life expectancy is reportedly close to 80, and some reports have it higher, in the neighborhood of 82.

These stats prove that it really is 'game on'; let us not hide from the facts and let us become proactive, accountable, and see the need for increased fundraising for Alzheimer's research. Bringing this into the mainstream of consciousness will assist in finding treatment and give us a game plan. Improving our QOL through preemptive lifestyle is imperative.

Cognitive brain health is achievable; follow Dr. Doriaswamy's advice which is, "eat your fruits and vegetables, exercise, don't be afraid to try new activities and be a social butterfly. Your brain will really thank you." Awareness and accountability will make a huge difference!

Remember we call all of this "Bounce"!

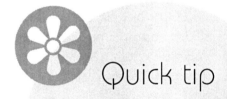

Quick tip

A well-hydrated person has the capacity to exercise 33% more than someone who is not.

40: Movement—The "Bounce Program"

I work out, not to regain my youth (frankly, my youth and young adulthood were a struggle); rather I want to create the mature me...to become a new and better person. This dwelling on the past, the longing for what is gone is a mirage in the desert and really serves no purpose. Frankly, studies have shown that mentally, you are at your pinnacle past 45 and on, so my mindset is to match the wisdom. And the great thing is, the more I focus on doing the small things (eating better, avoiding the bad nutrition, exercising), the better my mind seems to be working; I truly feel that the doctor's advice is right on, that for me it is all about these small steps. I mean, if you need encouragement to move more check this out:

Studies have shown, along with interviews I have conducted (Drs. Bartzokis, and Kramer come to mind) that aerobic movement (exercise) may reduce your chances of developing dementia and Alzheimer's, slowing the progress of their onset and potentially the progression if and when it starts. That neurogenesis and neuroplasticity are enhanced by movement, by which the chemistry of your brain is affected and enhanced, which is a completely positive occurrence. Research done at the Mayo Clinic analyzed approximately 1,600 papers on movement (exercise) and brain health, and they conclude that "you make a very compelling argument for exercise as a disease-modifying strategy to prevent dementia and mild cognitive impairment." I can say for a fact that without my exercise routine, not only would I not have finished undergrad and graduate school, but I may not have lived past my 48th birthday.

These little changes, the incremental improvements, add up over time to a new you. Forget the mindset of the fountain of youth—how about the fountain of health and longevity, which gives you the optimal QOL you are capable of achieving? I had to figure out my compelling 'why', the story, which led to the realization that brain health was so similar to my profession. I know that this drive to succeed, to help many use my story, comes from a power bigger than myself, much, much bigger. I keep hearing "Follow through; don't quit; don't give up." Sharing is where it is we are at, my friends.

I had this feeling that I needed to call this activities section something. I need a name for our program, so all of a sudden I thought of "Bounce". Just bounce. It fits; it is spontaneous, and it is adaptable to anyone and anywhere, sort of like all of us: "adaptable". So bounce it is, it is better to be creative and different; God knows we all are, right? Your fun may be one thing and mine might be another. Bounce is our mindset with movement; it is fun, always changing, never rigid. Be open to change, and your routine never becomes stale; use new challenges as an opportunity to explore—think of it as recess for grownups. So now what? Where from here? What time is it, everyone? Did you know that people who stay active as they age can slow down brain erosion? Studies are showing that in recent retirees, those who "bounced" (exercised) maintained nearly the same level of blood flow in their brains after several years, and that inactive people showed a significant *decrease*. If your brain is not growing, if the neurogenesis stops, than it is dying, which exacerbates cognitive decline. Movement and "Bounce" is the preventive medicine; we all age, and there is something we can do to increase our odds—it is exciting to think about.

It's that time where for some of us, our children have finally left the nest and are off at college starting their new lives. But while they're starting new lives, what are we, the parents, to do? Beginning to adjust to the "empty nest syndrome" can be difficult at first, but in the long run there are lots of benefits to an empty nest. No more mountains of clothes piled up from soccer games and school uniforms. Although it can sometimes be lonely without your kids in the house, now you can get back to the days when it was just you and your wife/husband, being "college kids" yourselves. It's now your turn to have some fun...again! Here are a few ideas of some ways to cope with "the empty nest syndrome", starting over, college and Math 106.

Math 106

Bodybuilding and college for a boomer, now that was an odd combination; looking back through the lens of a writer I see the complementary focuses of the huge "how".

It was the time-management techniques!

In the Fall of 2002, I had been back in the gym for a couple of years and physically, things were just okay. I had made a switch to an afternoon gym workout routine because I had discovered that after Sandy and I had married, the morning sessions I had become accustomed to were not conducive to a happy home. Namely, she needed some assistance with Lauren (our youngest), getting her off to elementary school; at that point, it was fine; however, the slow climb back up the weight mountain had begun, unbeknownst to me. A relationship and marriage take these things called teamwork and cooperation!

If I had known then what I now know, in regard to eating the correct foods, portion control, timing, healthy fats and the whole body building HyMEP, I am sure everything would have been totally cool. However, that was in the future and I was still under the impression that you could follow my modified Bill Phillips' "Body for Life" plan and have the free day and subsist.

Well, notice how I said "modified", and this is where the problem started to recur. My own modification, and I believe many people fall into this trap—the rollercoaster of fatness, extended the "Body for Life" free day into a couple of days, and then into three days, and that was a total killer for anyone trying to maintain any semblance of weight management. Calories in, calories out, it is simple addition. In addition, I had not realized the negativity of soft drinks, even diet soft drinks, fast food, prepared food and on and on; I think you get the picture. Clueless? Yep! Uninformed nutritionally, that was a given. But luckily, now happily married and back in college, my personal dynamics had changed, a lot!

So, getting back to the fall of 2002, I started an undergraduate class called "Math 106", which, if you have not had a math course in say, uhm, 20 years, can be a little bit daunting. This one was more than daunting; it was horrible! It was another of those University "weeder" classes, and in the same amphitheater classroom as my very first class, with 400 or so freshman. I was, again, against the wall of academia; it was like going in front of the firing squad. My professor, who was a very kind but very strict much older instructor, did not give off an air of anything other than strictly business. This was another of those second-guessing times in your life when you really think about your "why". As in, "Why in the hell am I torturing myself with this stuff?" Time management, learning how to learn, figuring it out—this was not going to be easy, and I needed a strategy. So I decided that I had to put in as much time as I possibly could; it was my own Chinese water torture.

It's called the lunch-time math help room.

This is where you go as a know-nothing (no offense to the traditional students) to learn material, tutoring at its finest. That in conjunction with spending every hour at home that I could muster working on problems was the only way, and it sucked! I found a student undergrad advisor in the help room who had pity on me, and with his help, and I am talking every day for a semester at lunch time, we worked on problems. It gave me much admiration for this young man and our younger generation of millennials, because without him I was toast. I found out after the fact from my professor that the assistance this young man provided me, the kindness, the love and the being there, prompted him to go into the teaching profession, true story.

Basically, I told myself that the workouts, the luxury of my lunchtime workouts were not important; I think, deep down, it was partially an excuse. "I don't have the time", and I was a self-absorbed, self-indulgent infantile; excuses are like assholes—everyone has one and they all stink. I built my own and I was the biggest. If I was going to suffer, well by God so was everyone else; what a dick I was.

Payback: 25 pounds, the understanding that I was selfish, and that if I was ever to amount to anything I had to quit making excuses and just get it done. Math 106 taught me some valuable lessons, lifelong lessons! Sandy put up with my arrogant 'baby-ness', and my children, for some unknown reason, still loved me, and I actually did pretty well in the course, scoring an unreal 3.0; my professor was very impressed. So what is the point of this story to our movement/fitness section of the book?

Time management and giving to yourself the release of stress through movement, which I now know that if I had just figured out, or stuck to a smaller program, would have been very helpful to my not regaining those 25 pounds.

Because, let me tell you, my numbers went through the roof, which started my journey to getting everything back, which in retrospect really was a good thing for me, in some fat goofy way. Remember how, in the behaviors section of the book, I did the informal survey of students and staff who were dedicated gym rats? This whole Math 106 experience started that mindset. And the biggest thing that came out of this experience was confidence. I now knew in my heart that my wife really did love me for all of my faults, and that was of paramount importance (because, frankly, she should have kicked my sorry ass to the curb), and if I could make it through this one course, this one mountain, then I could accomplish anything.

That, my friends, lead us to the next phase: finding what works for you, and getting it done! Let's talk fun and funk.

41: Put the fun into funk

So what is fun, this simple three-letter word? Is it an action, a state of mind, a belief or memory? Is it just losing control and letting your inhibitions jump out the window? Sometimes the things we take for granted are the most elusive. So what is fun, and how do we capture its essence—the yin?

When Sandy and I coached girls' softball, we learned that one of the things that you try and do in team sports to be successful is instill a love for what you are doing. And the only way you can do that is by instilling that intrinsic feeling of enjoyment. Ask yourself if you like what you are doing.

Some team sports are really pretty boring, when you come right down to it. It is not always the competition that makes the competitor, the athlete, want to spend the time improving their skill. A lot of the time it is the socialization that brings the player to the field, because we are social animals who like to do things in a group, for enjoyment and fun.

Getting six- and seven-year-old girls to want to play softball is a challenge; herding butterflies might be easier. Any time you assemble a diverse group of children and try and teach them a thinking, skill game like softball (many team sports are thinking games), you have a daunting task, so what to do when the girls lose their attention in like two minutes of standing on a field? You build on the enjoyment factor; you get them to like it. You have fun.

It will be those memories that you build that will always exist in your mind, and as an adult you will need to pull that feeling out when you get busy with other activities. Put the fun in funk; now we are setting the stage for improving our QOL.

People will do what they enjoy doing, and if you don't enjoy the activity then chances are you are not going to do it. That has to be one of my most profound statements ever(sarcasm)! Even if you know that something is good for you, if your mindset is negative, it's not happening.

Becoming more active and losing your inhibition, finding what provides amusement or enjoyment specifically, is the key to this chapter.

Back to the softball team first, though; if you can herd those little butterflies and make them a winning, fun group, now you have cracked the code, and you have to capture that essence and share it. Read on.

Enjoyment and boisterous activity is a natural behavior; we are born with that running and jumping desire and we are taught as youngsters to control it. That in itself is the problem—the control factor, the "don't do that" mentality. That is what gets in our way of letting the hair down. Remember the section on the NET, negative energy is a killer.

Being aware of what we like or love to do is what we need to find, that experience, the feeling that is so deeply suppressed in all of us. What is it you like to do? And why don't you do it more often? Or maybe you need to try some new activities to put the fun in your funk, something outside the comfort zone.

You see, the kids that I coached wanted to learn something new, but were afraid at first. Sure, but that didn't stop them, because I figured out the motivation side of group activity quickly, basically just pulling from my own memories as a kid playing sports, what worked, and went for it.

Fun is not brain surgery, or is it?

Socialization is one of the keys, finding the constructive environment, something that works for you that is not harmful to your body. As we grow up we get so busy, and the essence is pushed farther into our memories, to the point where we can't even remember what it feels like to have that boisterous exhibition of behavior, fun. I believe that is why we have such a problem with substance abuse; it is fun through chemistry, and that is why drugs and alcohol are so addictive—they release the dopamine, the neurotransmitter in your brain that will make you feel good.

Pure Michigan—Dave Lorenz

Dave Lorenz[42] has become a regular on "Boomers Rock", our radio show; he was really my first regular guest and has remained with me ever since. I had this idea of integrating travel into the talk show, because I know that finding quality vacations at affordable prices is really important, plus I figured in a self-serving way I could learn about cool spots and maybe do some remotes, promote the resort and visit, a win-win.

Dave Lorenz works for Travel Michigan as the manager of the Public & Industry Relations department within the Michigan Economic Development Corporation; he is the all-knowing sage as far as travel ideas. I had the idea to help promote my home state, so I dropped an email to the marketing arm of our tourism department, "Pure Michigan", and Dave responded, setting up our new friendship. I have to say, it has been a huge hit and he is a total pro for talk show content.

Being a team sport person for most of my life, I have never really been into the hunting-gathering outdoors stuff, not in the least, Dave has enlightened me as far as new adventure goes, and the quality of memory building you can accomplish through some of his suggestions, for example. We have talked about kayaking, canoeing, mountain biking, hiking, dune buggy riding, horseback riding, hunting and fishing, just to name a few things. We have an ice-climbing adventure on the books, and he is going to set it up so I can take myself in the cold and experience a new adventure.

He came up with the term "Cross-generational", which I have stolen and now use on the talk show all the time. This kind of activity, this "cross-generational" fitness is a perfect way to find new things to do as a family or with a group of people from all different age groups. It is a magnificent way to incorporate movement into your life and build new relationships, bonds and memories. I just love the whole concept and it fits our fun into funk.

Many of these ideas can be very cost effective, and extremely fun. I mean, if you ever want the thrill of dune buggy riding, along the water, in a very safe and wholesome family day, you could always visit the "Mac Woods" dune rides in northern Lower Michigan; getting into the outdoors with your children and/or grandchildren is what it is all about.

You realize that being around people, socializing, talking, and having fun releases serotonin, a neurotransmitter that is vital to our mood, learning and self-esteem. Serotonin is called the "policeman" of our brain, quelling overactive, out-of-control responses in a wide range of brain systems. Funk and remove the 'K', having fun and returning to your past/childhood and the beginner's mind; never lose the fun. Tap into it; letting go will always live inside all of us—it just needs to be rekindled. Think positive, build on it slowly and see what happens.

We were all young once and I truly feel that it is not regaining our youth that is the key to achieving that QOL, it's having fun, while using all of our knowledge and skills to enjoy it for what it is—just simple fun. I mean, do not get me wrong, I had some great times as a kid and teenager, plenty, but it is the now that we live in and enjoying what we do is the key to making the best of all of our situations. Without the fun it really is funk, right?

When we were children, yes, I remember, and I know you do too, there were things like a city-sponsored sort of a day camp at the local parks. I am sure many of you had this type of experience during the summer, because remember this was before cable TV and way, way before the internet came along and made everyone's life better... uhm, yeah. Anyway, remember those summer days? I certainly do and here is the rub—all of this has vanished, like the dinosaurs, extinct. Now you have arranged camps, or expensive week-long immersion-type situations that are really expensive. What to do, what to do.

We live in a beautiful home with a great park/elementary school directly behind our house, a really great place with a fantastic play set, swings, ball diamond, the whole nine yards; I mean really awesome. Attached to the school/park grounds is a large area of trees (I still call them woods), where you could build forts, hang out, pretend, and basically have a blast. The problem is I only rarely see kids playing out there (except in a structured environment like soccer), and when we do see kids they are usually older kids.

The point I am trying to make is this—unstructured play is a thing of the past, and I believe it is really hurting our kids and adults as well.

Putting the fun into funk is a concept that needs to be branded, or at least shared with all of our kids. Back in the dark ages (when we boomers were little), playing ball in the street, pickup games of hoop, shagging flies, playing 500—it was all part of growing up, and we need it back, badly. Structure has changed everything, and too much planning is overkill.

Play dates—where the heck did that come from?

I talk a lot on the radio show about "cross-generational fitness" (remember I stole it from Dave Lorenz); I know, a fancy term that covers a lot of ground, but in all simplicity it is getting outside and experiencing life with our kids. My dad used to play football in the street with us boys all the time. You get out there and play catch, throw the football around and before you know it you got a neighborhood game going on; those were the days, the days before iPods, laptops, and the internet. As I have read, "motion is lotion"; that is a cool metaphor and it is vastly underrated. It really is about getting outside and just having fun.

Unstructured fun and the value of play, spontaneous activity; when did everything have to become so planned? When was the last time you just said to your son or daughter let's go for a bike ride? Or let's go and play catch, or go for a run, or hike in the woods. Our society has become so busy, so structured, that we have to make an appointment with our own kids to do something spontaneous. Who is going to teach them the importance of this invaluable skill: making it up as we go along? Do you remember just jumping on your bike in the morning and disappearing? Mom saying, "Be home when the street lights come on." Do you remember some of those things Mom used to say, that at the time seemed ridiculous and now they turn out to be so true?

I did another informal survey on these sayings on my Facebook account one day looking for these sayings; let's see if you remember any of these:

"I TOLD YOU SO"

Mind your "p's" and "q's!" Whatever that is??

It only takes once to get pregnant.

My grandmother would say, "God's last name is not 'Damn'"

Fight nice, kids!

Don't try it because you just might like it.

If you can't say anything nice, don't say anything at all.

The first 90 years are the hardest; after that it's a breeze. (Referring to marriage)

Treat others as you would want to be treated.

Choose your battles.

I brought you in to this world, and I will take you out.

If you don't wipe that silly look off your face I'll do it for you.

The faster you go, the behinder you get.

'Can't' never did anything.

Everything happens for a reason.

Cut that out or I'll knock you into next week! Or I'll knock your heads together, or I'll box your ears!

Don't you roll your eyes at me!

All. The. Time.

No pain no gain.

The bigger they are the harder they fall.

Practice makes perfect.

Fun into funk can come in many flavors, and for us boomers, isn't that sweet? As I was thinking about this chapter and pulling thoughts together, more and more fun thoughts just kept coming. For example, fun group exercise classes.

Group exercise?

I have to say that before I had my epiphany, my thought on a group class was absolutely zero; never done it and really didn't have any inclination. So you see, trying new things is really a good thing, because frankly, this is what I have personally done in the last three years. Check this out

First it started with my friend and trainer Tom Mitchell convincing me to try his Spin class. First off I thought to myself, "What the hell is Spinning and why do I want to try this?" Well, for the know-nothing that I was at the time, Spinning is a high-intensity cycling class done in a group setting to music, loud music, and you basically follow the instructor through a series of settings on the stationary bike. Up hills, speed work, slow speed, standing, sitting—I thought, "No big deal, right?" Uhm, wrong.

Spinning is the type of cardio workout that will just crush you if you try and keep up with the other members in the class. Oh, did I mention that the class was at MSU and had like 25 college students, three faculty, and the average age was 21? Yeah! Tom Mitchell, my buddy Vennie Gore I were the oldest people in the class and Mr. Mitchell, yes he is a machine, so I had a long way to go. But you know what? It was fun! Yes, a bitch and a half, but fun.

Remember fun into funk, right?

The best thing about spin is the ability to just go at your own pace and no one really cares, so you can ease your way into the water so to speak, and not drown. I did see some college men, trying to impress the new girlfriend, crash and burn, trying to be Mr. Macho. Halfway through the class, they blow chunks, or almost pass out. You really want to stay within yourself for this bad boy. Full out Spinning is not for the rookies; just get used to the whole situation. You are only competing with yourself, but I still highly recommend this class; it rocks.

Yoga

Yoga is becoming such a mainstream group class now, and I have done this a few times. My goal is to incorporate yoga into my routine, and there is a new studio opening. Sandy and I are going for it. For those of us who need the stretching, say lifters, Yoga is for you. I have modified my daily ritual to incorporate a hybrid half-hour early-morning yoga session, with a warm-up on the bike and a small amount of resistance. It is a good start; warm-ups for the day work well and don't have to be insanely complicated. Less is better, anyway.

Listen to this:

If you are wondering and/or looking for that new thing, new class, or just new exercise philosophy, yoga can provide you with many health benefits without the undue strain of some other types of fitness regimens. Some of the bennies of Yoga (which did originate in India like 5,000 years ago) are particularly good for boomers and seniors. Why? Because Yoga generates body motion without causing that undue strain of other types of fitness programs; it is completely different than other forms of exercise. Here are some general Yoga benefits:

- Sharpens the mind and helps with concentration

- Is a natural body relaxer

- Chronic stress patterns are relieved

- Relieves muscle strain and refreshes the body

- And, of course, the mental relaxation is incredible

Yoga is a great program for people of all ages and fitness levels. It really can be very physically demanding for athletes (especially lifters and body builders), but it can be practiced at your own pace in a gentle way. Some studies have shown that boomers participating in Yoga activities experience better sleep, increased strength (without the muscle strains), and improved flexibility. If you suffer from rheumatoid arthritis, Yoga can enhance and increase your QOL, our purpose with this book and the radio show, right? Diabetics who followed a 40/40 routine (sessions and minutes per class) had improved fasting blood sugar, and hypertension sufferers saw a decrease in blood pressure, cholesterol and triglycerides, along with feeling more relaxed. In addition, more studies have shown that Yoga has helped people manage weight, stress and anxiety, plus chronic pain.

I had the pleasure of interviewing Yogi Cameron on "Boomers Rock", and his gentle demeanor, thoughts on diet and the mental aspects of Yoga, were simply amazing. His book *The Guru in You*[43] is phenomenal and will take you into his personal journey of transformation from superstar fashion model to becoming the Yoga master to Hollywood types like Madonna and Ellen DeGeneres.

This group class will put the fun back into funk for sure!

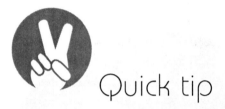

Quick tip

As we age (after 30), we naturally lose muscle, unless you train with resistance or weight bearing exercises. If you maintain the same eating habits, foods, timing, etc., you will inevitably gain weight.

42: Chronic Pain

Pain affects more Americans than diabetes, heart disease and cancer combined. As recently as 20 years ago, chronic pain was dismissed a purely psychological—a symptom of suspected higher mental illness—and treated with a non-caring attitude. Today, according to many doctors, pain is recognized as a disease.

Pain is an intricate relationship between the neurotransmitters in your brain and your spinal cord. The body produces natural painkillers like serotonin, norepinephrine and opioid-like chemicals.

People with chronic pain are twice as likely to suffer from depression and anxiety as those who are not suffering. You enjoy life less; your mind and spirit are affected.

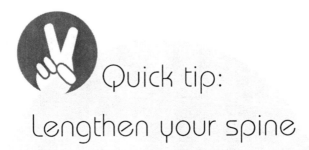

Quick tip:

Lengthen your spine

"Think of your vertebrae as an Oreo Cookie—there's a bone, then the squishy center (the disc), and then another bone," says Dr. James Rudolph, M.D., an assistant professor at Harvard medical school. "As those discs lose water over time, your spine compresses."

To slow the process, improve your posture. Standing straighter and using good form when exercising can make a difference in the long run, and help strengthen our tree trunk (core), avoiding chronic pain and potential injury. In some cases, exercise and stretching have been shown to help alleviate pain, and acupuncture has helped many. Meditation may benefit chronic pain sufferers by reducing the emotional stress. The settling, relaxed state has been indicated to reduce stress. In addition, the American Chronic Pain Association (theacpa.org) has a five-minute relaxation exercise that can be effective at helping you let go of the physical stress that exacerbates pain.

The chart below depicts the number of chronic pain sufferers compared to other major <u>health conditions.</u>

Condition	Number of Sufferers	Source
Chronic Pain	116 million people	Institute of Medicine of The National Academies
Diabetes	25.8 million people (diagnosed & estimated undiagnosed)	American Diabetes Association
Coronary Heart (heart attack and chest pain)	16.3 million people 7.0 million people	American Heart Association
Cancer	11.7 million people	American Cancer Society

The Burden of Pain on Everyday Life

The total annual incremental cost of health care due to pain ranges from $560 billion to $635 billion (in 2010 dollars) in the United States, which combines the medical costs of pain care and the pecuniary costs related to disability days and lost wages and efficiency.

More than half of all hospitalized patients experienced pain in the last days of their lives and, although therapies are present to alleviate most pain for those dying of cancer, research shows that 50-75% of patients die in moderate to severe pain. An estimated 20% of American adults (42 million people) report that pain or physical discomfort disrupts their sleep a few nights a week or more[44].

The tree analogy and chronic pain

As I said, this activities section is not going to be an exercise-specific kind group of chapters. I wanted more of a seed planting, get-you-thinking-about-the-steps kind of chapter. I do want to go back and touch on a couple of things that we had covered earlier in the book, so let's revisit the concept of "Neurogenesis".

First though, I want to share with you my tree analogy:

It took me a long time, most of my adult life, when I actually got back into the gym, to understand what is actually important, how to be efficient, and to not feel like a total dumbass going back into the fitness center after a long layoff. When you really start to see the benefits of your new "activities" program, (see how I am staying away from specifically calling this "exercise"?), core is king. Cardio movement is much better and easier to sustain when you understand the benefits of core, and with this in mind think back to neurogenesis and the dentate gyrus.

Cardio movement will make your dentate gyrus love you, and that is a really good thing.

Your dentate gyrus is a small section of your brain, and recently has been gathering a lot of attention, as well it should. It is a small section of your hippocampus, an area critical for memory, which as we age is going to be important to our state of mind, and cognitive awareness. I hate it when I can't find my keys, or forget someone's name, and so with movement you help your brain stay young, and remember where you parked the car.

I can tell you that there is no doubt in my mind that my activities program has increased my state of well-being, that I feel the best I have ever felt in my life, and I know that it is the activities program that I follow.

Now the tree analogy (digress, the story of my life).

In my world of metaphors, analogies, and being a longtime fan of all of the '60s television sitcoms and cartoons, my mind always gravitates toward the drawing of the picture in my mind. I think it has to be "Gilligan's Island" and the professor constantly creating and inventing some outrageous device from a coconut shell or a piece of seaweed. He could dream up the most outlandish of the outlandish, and they still never were rescued from the island.

Mindset and mapping, deep metaphors and goofy analogies; so here is the tree—I think you will like it.

The tree analogy is something akin to a giant willow tree we had in our backyard as a kid, a huge beautiful tree. I like to share this with everyone in the gym, or anyone who will listen; I think it is that important to think about. The beautiful tree: think hard about the big full tree casting shade, full of leaves in the summer, a spot to rest against or look at from a distance in all of its magnificence; you could see its towering silhouette for miles. Can you see it?

Your body is like that tree, a wonderful creation, God's gift to you and you alone. You maintain the essence of your own tree, feeding it, watering it, growing. Many people would like their tree to be pretty, look great from a distance, strong limbs, that bodybuilder symmetry, not all bulky and deformed, even and firm. The problem lies in our core, our trunk so to speak, where not much effort goes into the 27 muscles that make up our core; the focus is on what you can see, maybe the six-pack. Are you getting the visual?

The tree is only as strong as its trunk, its core, the area that supports your limbs and the area that supplies all of the nutrients to your leaves. It all revolves around what you can see, your visual perception, and that is where the tree analogy is so critical. The core holds all of the critical weight and stability of our tree; it is our support mechanism. If the entire trunk of your tree is weak, than you could have a beautiful outline; however, at the first inclement weather your magnificent tree is vulnerable—this is when we need that strength to carry us through, the stability to endure.

"From a small seed a mighty trunk may grow."
~Aeschylus

Back injuries (been there, don't want to go back) and chronic pain are major influencers of our QOL, and our understanding for strengthening our tree's trunk (core) is a major factor in avoiding and/or limiting the debilitating effects.

Your core is the key component to your body; your tree trunk (core) is a strong wind away from crashing to the ground. Back injuries are cited as the most common reason for absenteeism in the general workforce after the common cold.

It is estimated that about 70 to 85 percent of adults experience a back injury in their lifetime, and about 10 percent will suffer a re-injury, leaving some seven million either partially or severely disabled. Lower back pain accounts for some estimated 93 million workdays lost. Nationally, back injuries cost this country more than $100 billion annually in medical bills, disability and lost productivity at work. If surgery is involved, the cost for claims increases significantly to $40,000 per injury or higher. Lower back pain is one of the costliest health problems in the U.S., and what starts at your back can eat at your entire being[45].

43: Motion is lotion

Overuse and underuse injuries: Finding our balance

The oldest of our senior citizens grew up in an age of much less exercise than their parents. They were among the first Americans to have access to such labor-saving devices as washing machines, clothes dryers, power lawn mowers, which include riding mowers, and other time-saving devices.

The foundation was being built toward the sedentary American.

Our bodies were designed to move—to stretch, to run, walk and jump. Remember playing outside until the streetlights came on? For some it is unfortunate that by age 50 just getting out of bed is a major chore. This can be attributed to our sedentary lifestyle, which can lead us to depression, fatigue, low adrenal function and lack of quality sleep, ugh!

Technology now has evolved to the point of instant gratification, due to the internet, online shopping, and computing. Telecommuting, staying at home and working through a remote desktop application is widely used. We are more advanced technologically, but less healthy than our grandparents, all due to lack of movement and physical labor.

Here is more information from our buddy Dr. Art Kramer. He was studying the sedentary, inactive, and immobile; "We chose couch potatoes," he stated as the study's lead author. The 214 healthy adults hadn't been involved in any physical exercise for the previous five to 10 years. "Indeed, most of our subjects hadn't done any formal exercise for more like 30 or 40 years."

One group took long walks three times a week, and the other only did gentle toning and stretching exercises using weights. Walkers, who completed an hour-long loop around the university, improved significantly in the mental tests, as well as being fitter; an improvement of only five to seven percent in cardio-respiratory fitness led to an improvement of up to 15 percent in mental tests. The non-walkers, however, did not gain any benefits for their brains.

"We see selective cognitive benefits which accompany improvement in aerobic fitness," says Kramer. Although benefits were not obvious in every type of test, improvements were clearly attributable to the aerobics workout. Even beyond age 70, cardiovascular exercise can improve memory and reasoning skills. "People who have chosen a lifetime of relative inactivity can benefit mentally from improved aerobic fitness. It's never too late."

It has been reported that the average American watches television for five hours a day, which equates to over 70 days a year. A recently published research study by the Journal of the American Medical Association indicated that the long hours watching television were associated with many lack-of-movement ailments. The value of exercise and movement is at a premium, with overweight issues (due to a sedentary lifestyle), bordering on obesity, leading to a massive wave of health-related issues, for example diabetes, heart disease, and osteoarthritis. Motion can truly be lotion!

Osteoarthritis

Osteoarthritis afflicts 30 million in the U.S. and is growing; we must take care of our bones and joints, and strengthening muscles will help stabilize our joints. Osteoarthritis is the most common type of arthritis, affecting nearly 30 million Americans. The degenerative joint disease is characterized by a breakdown of cartilage— the tissue that cushions the end of bones and allows them to move smoothly. Typically, osteoarthritis occurs in hips, hands, knees, lower back, and neck.

A recent study conducted at Penn State College of Medicine found that patients who lost weight but received no other treatments for knee osteoarthritis experienced improvements in quality of life, the ability to perform day-to-day tasks and their capacity to participate in sports activities. "Weight loss is probably the number one factor for osteoarthritis pain," notes Nathan Wei, M.D., Director of the Arthritis Treatment Center in Frederick, Maryland. He stresses the importance of making dietary changes and exercising.

Movement is a key component to alleviating osteo-arthritis. Unfortunately, osteoarthritis pain makes it difficult to exercise, but studies show that exercise strengthens muscles and tissues around the cartilage, and can significantly reduce inflammation and pain. "Exercise is a big part of the lifestyle change that's necessary to deal with OA," says Noels Carlson, M.D., Assistant Professor in the Department of Orthopedics and Rehabilitation at Oregon Health and Sciences University. "It's a key to losing weight."

Low-impact movement can help assuage symptoms, such as aquatics, cycling, and walking, which can build strength and burn calories. But jumping into an exercise program that is not properly thought out can defeat your purpose, causing overuse injuries.

I battled through elbow tendonitis for months after the bodybuilding show. My excitement toward reaching the bucket list goal was achieved, but because I became such a training fiend I suffered through the pain, while it could have been avoided. As you reach your exercise goals you will feel much more energy and your enthusiasm will build; don't let overuse or overtraining sidetrack your effort; motion is lotion, and balance is bliss.

Be aware and be careful; at this point in our lives it really is about quality of life, not quantity of pushups.

"Wolff's Law"

Bone is laid down where needed and reabsorbed where not needed, according to demands.

Wolff's law is a theory developed by the German anatomist-surgeon Julius Wolff (1836–1902) in the 19th century, which states that bone in a healthy person or animal will adapt to the loads it is placed under. If loading on a particular bone increases, the bone will remodel itself over time to become stronger to resist that sort of loading. For example:

- Weightlifters often display increases in bone density in response to their training.

- The racquet-holding arm bones of tennis players become much stronger than those of the other arm. Their bodies have strengthened the bones in their racquet-holding arm since it is routinely placed under higher-than-normal stresses.

- Astronauts who spend a long time in space will often return to Earth with weaker bones, since gravity hasn't been exerting a load on their bones. Their bodies have reabsorbed much of the mineral that was previously in their bones.

- Martial artists who strike objects with increasing intensity (or of increasing hardness), display increases in bone density in the striking area; this process is termed 'cortical remodeling' (Wolff's law).

- Running 30 miles or more per week makes frame problems likely; lower-impact cardio movement is recommended.

Strengthening your quadriceps can reduce the risk of osteoarthritis by 30 percent; chair squats are a good example of quad-building exercises. In addition, studies show that walking daily can lower risks of heart attack and stroke by 20 to 33 percent.

Two types of muscle fibers in the body: Fast-twitch and slow-twitch

There are two types of muscle fibers in your body: type I, or slow-twitch fibers, which contract slowly but have great endurance; and type II, or fast-twitch fibers, which contract quickly but have low endurance capacities. Use this analogy: slow-twitch muscles are long distance, the marathoner muscles, while the fast-twitch are explosive lifting muscles. Understanding both is important, as they have a synergistic symbiosis in our body.

Muscles drive metabolism, your furnace to the metabolic oven, and muscle loss is preventable. Muscles reach their maximum size by about the age of 25 in most people. At this point there is then about a 10 percent decrease between the age of 25 and 45, with a 45 percent shrinkage over the next 30 years. Why does so much muscle tissue disappear, and why does the degeneration accelerate after the age of 50? New research from Sweden has the answer. The main reason for the reduction is that the total number of cells in any particular muscle stays pretty constant until the age of 30, but then begins a steady decline. The fall-off is slow at first but increases dramatically after the age of 50. For example, if one of your muscles consisted of 100 cells (fibers) when you were 30, the muscle would probably still contain 90 to 95 fibers 20 years later, but the 'fiber count' would plummet to only 50 to 55 when you reached the age of 50.

A decrease in the size of type II (fast-twitch) explosive-lifter fibers plays a key role in the muscle-shrinking process, with individual fast-twitch fibers contracting by about 25 to 30 percent between the ages of 20 and 80. Interestingly though, the type I (slow-twitch), endurance marathon-maker muscle cells, either remain unchanged in size or can expand by up to 20 percent in individuals who remain very physically active as they get older. This therefore compensates for the loss of size of type II fibers. But what causes the fairly dramatic loss in muscle cell numbers, clinically referred to as "sarcopenia". Over time (especially after the age of 50), motor nerve cells in the spinal cord begin to deteriorate at a steady rate. The motor nerve cells are normally in close contact with muscle cells and tell the muscle fibers when to contract during physical activity. The deterioration of fast-twitch motor neurons, which leads to the decrease in muscle mass and strength, is called "aptosis" (cell death). In simplified terms it is the proverbial "use it or lose it" disease.

This connection between motor nerves, and their associated muscle cells, is also necessary to keep the muscle fibers alive. Therefore, as motor nerve cells die, the muscle cells to which they are attached also bite the dust. Recall the earlier topic of myelin, and passionate practice; it is always about the movement theory.

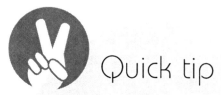

Quick tip

Build more muscle, as muscle burns more calories (5) than fat does (2). If you're over 40, you're losing a little muscle mass each year so weight-bearing exercises like lifting weights are needed to maintain or build muscle.

"Nothing lifts me out of a bad mood better
than a hard workout on my treadmill. It never
fails. Exercise is nothing short of a miracle."

~Cher

Resistance training: Positive effects

Fortunately, there's a positive side to the story. People
who participate in resistance training don't necessarily
halt the fiber-death process, but they can stop and even
reverse the reduction of size in the type II fibers (again I
iterate this, passionate practice, and myelin). Although
the number of muscle cells declines, type II (and sometimes even type I) fibers may get larger as a result of
strength training, leading to a potential advancement,
instead of a loss of total muscle tissue in the body. Since
the overall process of muscle atrophy (reduction) picks
up steam after the age of 50, strength training for people over 50 is especially critical. Fortunately, it's never
too late. Research demonstrates that even individuals
over the age of 80 can improve their muscles by participating in regular strength training workouts.

At 50 and older, exercise and movement are a tonic
with miraculous effects on mood and weight loss; energy levels can soar, and your quality of sleep is enhanced.
Exercise enhances and stimulates sensory and motor
cortices and maintains your brain's balance system. A
brutal workout is not necessary; just consistent natural
movement of your limbs works great, and simply walking works great. In addition, exercise and movement
boosts immunity, is a natural appetite suppressant, im-

proves your HDL (the good cholesterol), increases the release of pain-reducing endorphins, strengthens our bones (Wolff's law), improves our circulation and respiration, and lowers the chance of cardiovascular disease.

Our perpetual "Indian summer" of our lives should be a wonderful time of looking forward to continued growth; unfortunately for many our backs ache, our necks and shoulders are tight, our knees creak and our hips hurt; dang it! So without a plan, we are stuck. So, follow my lead, because if it can work for me it certainly can work for you. The sooner you begin to plant the seeds of change, small steps to improving your movement, nurturing your body and frame, the better the passage of time can be; you just gotta believe and start moving.

Call it looking forward to aging gracefully, giving you the best odds; *all of this talk of "reversing" the aging process plants the seed of looking backward, when we all have so much potential to look forward, if we do the right things. For example:*

Get regular medical exams and preventive health screenings: *Many diseases that can affect your health are highly treatable when detected early.*

Eat well: *Numerous studies indicate that a healthy diet can help you live longer and better. Eat foods that have lots of essential nutrients in proportion to their calories: whole grains, fresh vegetables and fruits and legumes.*

Keep physically active: *Aim for 30 minutes or more of exercise most days of the week. Benefits include weight control, improved blood circulation, increased muscle mass, greater flexibility, more endurance and improved balance.*

Use sun protection: *Sun exposure is responsible for much of the skin damage associated with aging and is the major risk factor for skin cancer.*

Avoid tobacco use: *Smoking is linked to various cancers, as well as to high blood pressure, heart disease, stroke and lung disease.*

Stay socially connected and intellectually curious: *Having strong ties to family and friends can buffer or reduce some health-related effects of aging and stress. Exercising your brain with classes, hobbies, reading and other mind-challenging activities can help you better maintain your memory.*

Limit alcohol: *More than one drink a day for women can increase the risk of cardio vascular disease, some cancers, and liver and pancreatic diseases. Alcohol can weaken your immune system, affect your cognitive abilities and increase your risk of falling.*

Part 4:

Grimoire

A Grimoire is a textbook of magical spells and recipes. I want to be very clear that what is listed is not magic, not at all. However, the results and changes I have experienced are in essence "Magical". I have struggled my entire life with weight, bad blood-work numbers, high blood pressure, cholesterol, triglycerides, you name it. The following information is what I do, and how I do it, and what got me into the best shape and health of my life. Ordinary guy, accomplishing the extraordinary.

It may not be magic, but it certainly is "Magical"!

The supplements, foods, eating plan and journal entries are all completely factual. What I wanted to accomplish is to give you value in this book by having an easy reference section, a place where you could look up the HyMEP and follow the lead and pick and choose; remember I have talked about "a la carte". This is it. If you decide to do one thing, great; it will make a difference. If you choose to to implement all, well hip-hip-hooray for you!

The one thing I never wanted to do with this book was ram information down someone's throat; it is always about choice—you choose—it is your QOL. This reference section is titled, "The Nitty Gritty".

44: The Nitty Gritty

I am going to list everything and define each item. You can start wherever you like, pick and choose; think of it as a buffet of good information and use the 'a la carte' method, because when it comes to the eating plan stuff, one size does not fit all.

Wheat grass

First thing every day is one ice cube of wheat grass in the morning with two to three ounces of warm water. One cube of wheat grass (we use the brand "Natures Wonder") may be sufficient for daily maintenance and supply of minerals, vitamins, amino acids and enzymes. We always do this first thing in the morning.

Benefits of wheat grass

WHEATGRASS JUICE...

...increases red blood cell count and lowers blood pressure. It cleanses the blood, organs and gastrointestinal tract of debris. Wheat grass also stimulates metabolism and the body's enzyme systems by enriching the blood. It also aids in reducing blood pressure by dilating the blood pathways throughout the body. Wheat grass stimulates the thyroid gland, correcting obesity, indigestion, and a host of other complaints.

Wheat grass restores alkalinity to the blood. The juice's abundance of alkaline minerals helps reduce over-acidity in the blood. It can be used to relieve many internal pains, and has been used successfully to treat peptic ulcers, ulcerative colitis, constipation, diarrhea, and other complaints of the gastrointestinal tract. Wheat grass is a powerful detoxifier, and liver and blood protector. The enzymes and amino acids found in wheat grass can protect us from carcinogens like no other food or medicine. It strengthens our cells, detoxifies the liver and bloodstream, and chemically neutralizes environmental pollutants. Wheat grass contains beneficial enzymes. Whether you have a cut finger you want to heal or you desire to lose five pounds...enzymes must do the actual work. The life and abilities of the enzymes found naturally in our bodies can be extended if we help them from the outside by adding exogenous enzymes, like the ones found in wheat grass juice. Don't cook it. We can only get the benefits of the many enzymes found in grass by eating/drinking it uncooked. Wheat grass offers the benefits of a liquid oxygen transfusion since the juice contains liquid oxygen. Oxygen is vital to many body processes: it stimulates digestion, promotes clearer thinking (the brain utilizes 25% of the body's oxygen supply), and protects the blood against anaerobic bacteria. Wheat grass is a superfood![46]

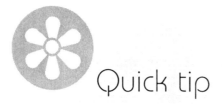

Quick tip

Wheat grass restores fertility
and promotes youthfulness.

Organic coconut oil, one tablespoon twice daily

As a healthy fat, a medium-chain fatty acid, I have become a complete believer in the benefits of coconut oil. I take one tablespoon in the morning and another when I return home from work. It works wonderfully as an appetite suppressant and gives me a nice combination of healthy fat, along with my juice and fish oil I do not ever need to snack after work.

The following are some of the benefits of organic coconut oil:

- Healthier hair

- Healthier skin

- Stress relief

- Maintaining cholesterol levels
- Weight loss
- Increased immunity
- Proper digestion and metabolism
- Reduced risk of heart diseases
- Reduced risk of diabetes

Fatty Acid Composition of Coconut Oil

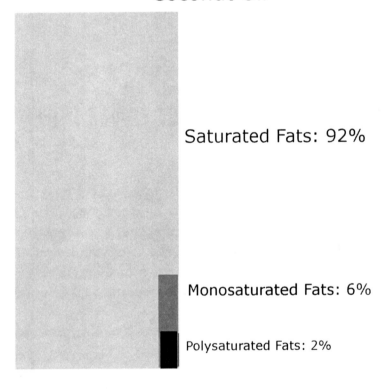

Saturated Fats: 92%

Monosaturated Fats: 6%

Polysaturated Fats: 2%

The benefits of coconut oil can be attributed to the presence of lauric acid, capric acid and caprylic acid (medium- and long-chain fatty acids), and its antimicrobial, antioxidant, antifungal, and antibacterial properties.

Composition of Coconut Oil:

- Coconut oil consists of more than 90 percent saturated fats with traces of a few unsaturated fatty acids, such as monounsaturated fatty acids and polyunsaturated fatty acids.

- The saturated fatty acids: Most of them are medium-chain triglycerides, which assimilate well.

- Lauric acid is the chief contributor, with more than 40 percent of the share, followed by capric acid, caprylic acid, myristic acid and palmitic acid.

- The polyunsaturated fatty acid: Linoleic acid.

- The monounsaturated fatty acid: Oleic acid.

- Vitamin E and Vitamin K, and minerals such as iron

Hair Care:

Coconut oil is one of the best natural 'foods' for hair. It helps in healthy growth of hair, providing shine. Coconut oil is extensively used in the Indian sub-continent for hair care. It is an excellent conditioner and helps in the re-growth of damaged hair. It also provides the essential proteins required for nourishing damaged hair. It is therefore used as hair care oil and used in manufacturing various conditioners and dandruff-relief creams. Coconut oil is normally applied topically for hair care.

Skin Care:

Coconut oil is an excellent massage oil for the skin, as well. It acts as an effective moisturizer on all types of skin, including dry skin. The benefit of coconut oil on the skin is comparable to that of mineral oil. Further, unlike mineral oil, there is no chance of having any adverse side effects on the skin with the application of coconut oil. Coconut oil therefore is a safe solution for preventing dryness and flaking of skin. It also delays wrinkles and sagging of skin, which normally become prominent with age. Coconut oil also helps in preventing premature aging and degenerative diseases due to its antioxidant properties.

Weight Loss

Coconut oil is very useful in reducing weight. It contains short- and medium-chain fatty acids that help in taking off excessive weight. It is also easy to digest and it helps in healthy functioning of the thyroid and enzymes systems. Further, it increases the body metabolism by reducing stress on the pancreas, thereby turning out more energy and helping obese and overweight people reduce their weight. Hence, people living in tropical coastal areas who eat coconut oil daily as their primary cooking oil are normally not fat, obese or overweight.

Digestion

Internal use of coconut oil occurs primarily as cooking oil. Coconut oil helps in improving the digestive system and thus prevents various stomach and digestion-related problems including irritable bowel syndrome.

The saturated fats present in coconut oil have antimicrobial properties and help in dealing with various bacteria, fungi, parasites, etc., that cause indigestion. Coconut oil also helps with absorption of other nutrients such as vitamins, minerals and amino acids.

Immunity:

Coconut oil is also good for the immune system. It strengthens the immune system, as it contains antimicrobial lipids, lauric acid, capric acid and caprylic acid, which have antifungal, antibacterial and antiviral properties.

The human body converts lauric acid into monolaurin, which is said to help in dealing with viruses and bacteria-causing diseases such as herpes, influenza, cytomegalovirus, and even HIV.

Liver:

The presence of medium-chain triglycerides and fatty acids helps in preventing liver diseases, as the substances are easily converted into energy when they reach the liver, thus reducing workload on the liver and also preventing the accumulation of fat.

Diabetes:

Coconut oil helps in controlling blood sugar, and improves the secretion of insulin. It also helps in effective utilization of blood glucose, thereby preventing and treating diabetes.

Dental Care:

Calcium is an important element present in teeth. Since coconut oil facilitates absorption of calcium by the body, it helps in getting strong teeth. Coconut oil reportedly stops tooth decay.

Finally

Coconut oil is often preferred by athletes and body-builders, and by those who are dieting. The compelling reason for this is that coconut oil contains fewer calories than other oils, its fat content is easily converted into energy, and it does not lead to accumulation of fat in the heart and arteries. Coconut oil helps in boosting energy and endurance, and enhances the performance of athletes[47].

Carlson's Fish Oil

Taken twice daily, one tablespoon per dose, I have found that not only is this great fish oil, but it also has been recommended by Dr. George Bartzokis of UCLA (as mentioned earlier in the book as our myelin expert), as one of the two he would recommend for preventing myelin deterioration. As Doctor George mentioned in our interview, some caplets or capsules may not have the attributes and testing for cold-water-derived fish oil as the Carlson's brand, and potentially could be contaminated with mercury.

Carlson's Fish Oil is rated among the best fish oils. The fish oil is recognized for a number of health benefits for the human body. It supplies the essential fatty acids in the body. The omega-3 fatty acids are effective to prevent a number of health problems. The most important omega-3 fatty acids found in fish oil are EPA and DHA. These are helpful to prevent the cardiovascular problems, inflammation, and colon health, and are effective for the proper development of brain. The fish oil of Carlson laboratory is rated among the best fish oils. This oil comes from the cold-water fishes that are found in deep Norwegian waters. It is refined and packed in Norway in order to make sure that the Carlson's Fish Oil is fresh.

Carlson's Fish Oil is extracted through a safe process that is called molecular distillation. In this process the oil is separated from the tissues by decreasing the temperature, and no chemical is used in this process. It is the best method as it not only ensures the freshness but also ensures that there is no chemical contamination in the oil. It is a scientifically proven process that removes every toxin and other contaminating elements found in crude oil extracted from the fleshes of the fish. All products from the Carlson Lab are tested regularly by using the AOAC international protocol to ensure freshness, potency and purity. The process of testing is performed by an independent, FDA-registered laboratory. It is determined in the test that the products are free of detectable levels of mercury, cadmium, lead, and PCBs, and many other contaminates. In addition to the EPA and DHA omega-3 acids, the fish oil is a good source of Vitamin E and some other vitamins as well. Carlson's Fish Oil comes in many different categories, offering choice to the customer[48].

The magic of juicing

One really great thing that we both do, Sandy and I, every day, is drink juice—not just any juice, our home-made freshly ground juice.

If Jack Lalanne can live to over 90 juicing his whole life there is something here, believe me. Actually I have recently added the juice-drinking to my afternoon routine, when I get home from work, as it really helps me get up for the radio show. We purchased a "Champion Juice Machine" and it is a beast—American-made and easy to clean. We juice at least once a week, sometimes a bit longer depending on our supply, but if we get low it is time to get busy. It takes us about a half an hour to make the juice (ingredients coming shortly), and Sandy's prep time, pre-cleaning and post-cleaning takes her about an hour, but however long it takes—we do it. Here is the standard list of our juice; it varies with the seasons, but the basic recipe is the same:

- Carrots
- Beets
- Apples
- Spinach
- Lemons

Those are the basic ingredients for every batch. We have added many different varieties of fruit and veggie, for example watermelon is awesome, and really adds smoothness to the juice. Any other veggie from our small garden when in season, for example cucumbers and tomatoes; melon has made its debut; really anything that is an edible vegetable or fruit can be added; the "Champion" has never met its match. As far as how much we make, it's normally around two gallons, but remember this has to be refrigerated, which is why we have an extra fridge in our garage to maintain freshness. Fresh juice has the live enzymes that are destroyed in store-purchased juice.

In the morning I also add two tablespoons of hemp protein powder and ground flax (descriptions coming up); fresh juice has very little fat or protein so these supplements have been working well. I have read that you should not store juice for longer than a few days; ours seems to maintain its freshness for a week refrigerated and in a sealed container. It really is about the desire to juice, like any other of our lifestyle changes, and the cost, around $10.00 per batch, seems reasonable.

Reasons to Juice

There are three main reasons why you will want to consider incorporating vegetable juicing into your optimal health program:

Juicing helps you absorb all the nutrients from the vegetables. This is important because most of us have impaired digestion as a result of making less-than-optimal food choices over many years. This limits your body's ability to absorb all the nutrients from the vegetables. Juicing will help to "pre-digest" them for you, so you will receive most of the nutrition, rather than having it go down the toilet.

Juicing allows you to consume an optimal amount of vegetables in an efficient manner. If you are a carb type, you should eat one pound of raw vegetables per 50 pounds of body weight per day. Some people may find eating that many vegetables difficult, but it can be easily accomplished with a quick glass of vegetable juice.

You can add a wider variety of vegetables in your diet. Many people eat the same vegetable salads every day. This violates the principle of regular food rotation and increases your chance of developing an allergy to a certain food. But with juicing, you can juice a wide variety of vegetables that you may not normally enjoy eating whole[49].

Nutiva Hemp protein

Another one of the many supplements that I found in prepping for the bodybuilding show is Nutiva hemp protein... yes, hemp. Bought as a powder online from Vitacost.com (all of our natural supplements are), I try to mix this plant-based protein into my juice (as I just mentioned), but also in any protein shake that I will occasionally make. This amazing plant is a protein powerhouse! I love the product made by Nutiva because it has 11 grams of protein and 14 grams of fiber per serving. Hemp protein powder is a raw, certified organic food that contains 37% protein, 43% fiber, and zero net carbs. It also comes with the benefit of 9% beneficial fats (omega-3,-6, and -9 plus GLA), chlorophyll, Vitamin E and iron. Overall, this to me is another superfood.

Ground Flax

Grinding of the flax seed with our little coffee grinder started long (several years) before the BB show prep. This one is all Sandy; she gets all the credit for this one. She was very close to being required to take some sort of cholesterol drug, but resisted and started using the flax in her yogurt. Grinding flax is easy and by far the best delivery of this supplement, and it is the most inexpensive and effective use. I add a tablespoon daily to my juice—that's it—don't overdue this one, no need. Most nutrition experts recommend ground flaxseed because your body is better able to digest it. Whole flaxseed may pass through your intestine undigested, which means you won't get all the health benefits. I have never used flaxseed oil, and have seen the cost at the health food store; it really is a tad on the pricey side.

Flaxseed is high in fiber, omega-3 fatty acids and phytochemicals called lignans. Flaxseed is commonly used as a laxative (to improve digestive health or relieve constipation). Both flaxseed and flaxseed oil have been used to help reduce total blood cholesterol and low-density lipoprotein (LDL, or "bad") cholesterol levels and, as a result, may help reduce the risk of heart disease. Although flaxseed oil also contains omega-3 fatty acids, it doesn't have the beneficial fiber that the seeds have. You can purchase raw flaxseed in bulk —whole or ground — at many grocery stores and health food stores. Whole seeds can be ground in a coffee grinder and then stored in an airtight container for several months. Refrigerating whole seeds may also extend their freshness.

Although the Institute of Medicine has not set a recommended daily intake for omega-3 fatty acids, it has established adequate intake amounts of between 1.1 and 1.6 grams a day for adults. One tablespoon of ground flaxseed provides 1.6 grams of omega-3 fatty acids[50].

Tips for including flaxseed in your diet:

- Add a tablespoon of ground flaxseed to your hot or cold breakfast cereal.

- Add a teaspoon of ground flaxseed to mayonnaise or mustard when making a sandwich.

- Mix a tablespoon of ground flaxseed into an 8-ounce container of yogurt.

- Bake ground flaxseed into cookies, muffins, breads and other baked goods.

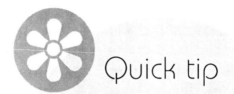

Quick tip

Be aware that buying flaxseed in bulk is by far our best option; I have seen many stores that sell pre-packaged seed for much more than the bulk health food option; watch your money and budget.

More ground flax tips

For the cost and benefits, ground flax has got to become a part of your daily routine. I can testify that it kept my wife from having to take cholesterol medication. Here are some other benefits from ground flax:

Cholesterol

Flax contains essential fatty acids, including omega-3 and omega-6, which help the body with many functions including controlling cholesterol levels and balancing good and bad fats.

Menopausal Symptoms

A poor diet can exacerbate menopausal symptoms, and a flaxseed supplement helps to balance estrogen levels and fill out an imbalanced, modern diet.

Cardiovascular Health, Weight Loss and Diabetes

Flaxseeds are an excellent source of all omega-3 essential fatty acids (including alpha-linoleic acids) that are critical for reducing the risk of heart disease and diabetes, as well as cancer. Omega-3s help balance blood sugar, boost metabolism and control appetite. Flax is known to help keep fats moving, as it emulsifies them in the body instead of storing them and keeps arteries from hardening.

Immune System and Inflammation

Flaxseeds are known to boost the immune system and relieve inflammation resulting from auto-immune diseases such as lupus, multiple sclerosis and rheumatoid arthritis.

Depression, Memory and Attention Deficit Disorder

The high levels of omega-3 and omega-6 fatty acids in flaxseeds help keep the brain, and its neural pathways, functioning properly so the brain does not have to over-compensate for inefficient links between cells.

Consuming flaxseeds should not encourage you to eat poorly or not exercise. While all of the health benefits of flaxseeds that are listed above have been evaluated for efficacy, flaxseeds are not a miracle product that will erase a multitude of sins from unhealthful living[51].

Cinnamon

Cinnamon has some surprising potential health benefits. Another of my daily additives, I don't think I can call this spice a supplement; however, used in conjunction with my "Bragg's Apple Cider Vinegar" (next on the list of the daily supplement routine), cinnamon has many outstanding benefits, which include:

Cinnamon has anti-inflammatory properties. Many of us eat lots of fried, fatty and processed foods, and these foods cause inflammation of our internal tissues and organs, and this inflammation has been linked to one of the most life-threatening diseases of our time – heart disease.

Cinnamon may actually help people with Type 2 diabetes control blood sugar levels, and may significantly lower LDL "bad" cholesterol, total cholesterol and triglycerides (fatty acids in the blood). A study was conducted by researchers from the US Department of Agriculture (USDA) in 2003 that showed that 60 people in Pakistan who had Type 2 diabetes, who ate 1 gram of cinnamon each day over a period of 40 days, experienced a significant decrease in their blood sugar levels, LDL cholesterol, total cholesterol and triglycerides.

A growing consensus among cardiologists pinpoints abnormal inflammation in artery walls as a root cause of atherosclerosis and coronary heart disease. Cinnamon could be a potential ally in our fight to decrease inflammation. Recall the interview I conducted with Dr. Lori Shemeck and our discussion of inflammation. With cinnamon's ability to regulate insulin it makes perfect and logical sense to try and incorporate small amounts into our diets, as Dr. Shemeck and I discussed sugar is a primary cause of inflammation[52].

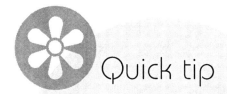

Quick tip

Since I have incorporated my healthy fats regimen on a consistent daily basis (Carlson's Fish Oil and virgin coconut oil), I rarely if ever take any ibuprofen, or similar OTC (over the counter) pain medication.

Bragg's Apple Cider Vinegar

"Bragg's Organic Apple Cider Vinegar is the #1 food I recommend for maintaining the bodies vital acid-alkaline balance and healthy digestion."

~Gabriel Cousens M.D.,
Author of *Conscious Eating*

My morning and afternoon routines (returning home from work, usually around 5:00ish) always involve a few key rituals, my routine. One of the key components of that routine is my "Bragg's Apple Cider Vinegar (ACV). I had seen the Bragg's vinegar at our local health food store and read about some of the natural healing powers of this product so I decided to try it; I bought the book, which explains many of its natural properties, and I was sold.

I had the pleasure to interview Patricia Bragg on "Boomers Rock" along with Barbara Gauene Muller (who has since become a guest host and great friend and inspiration to both Sandy and me). The Bragg family of all natural organic products has been around for 100 years as of this writing, and many notable fitness enthusiasts (including the legendary Jack Lalanne), were believers and advocates of the Bragg family of products. And now my family members are all believers and proponents of Bragg's ACV and its health benefits.

I drink approximately one ounce twice a day with about six ounces of water and a small amount of cinnamon; I find it to be an energy booster and great way to stabilize the PH level in my body. Here are some of the other benefits of Bragg's ACV:

- Promotes a youthful skin and vibrant healthy body

- Removes arterial plaque and is a natural detoxifier

- Fights germs, viruses, and bacteria naturally

- Helps regulate calcium metabolism

- Assists in women's menstrual cycles, relieving PMS and UTI

- Normalizes PH, and is a great source of potassium

- Helps in fighting arthritis and removes crystals and toxins from joints, tissues, and organs throughout the body

- Natural fat burner!

We use several other products in the Bragg family; they have so many it's hard to list them all, but we have personally used the "Liquid Amino Acid" salad dressing and the all-organic oil salad dressing. As I have a chance I will undoubtedly try more, as the products are cost effective and healthy, and any business that has been around for 100 years is pretty solid in my world.

If you are looking for a place to start the new you, this would be one I would consider first![53]

Spirulina and Chlorella

Another suggestion from my mentor and friend Chris Johnson (*On Target Living*), is absolutely an essential supplement to consider. I take (daily) 1000 mg of Spirulina, and 10 Chlorella tablets. The benefit of learning from knowledgeable people and taking their advice is critical. Just remember "small steps"!

Chlorella:

"Chlorella has been touted as the perfect whole food. Aside from being a complete protein and containing all the B vitamins, vitamin C, vitamin E, and the major minerals (with zinc and iron in amounts large enough to be considered supplementary), it has been found to

improve the immune system, improve digestion, de-
toxify the body, accelerate healing, protect against ra-
diation, aid in the prevention of degenerative diseases,
help in treatment of Candida albicans, relieve arthritis
pain and, because of its nutritional content, aid in the
success of numerous weight loss programs."[54]

Spirulina:

"Spirulina's predigested protein provides building material soon after ingestion, without the energy-draining
side effects of meat protein; its mucopolysaccharides
relax and strengthen connective tissue while reducing the possibility of inflammation; its simple carbohydrates yield immediate yet sustained energy; its GLA
fatty acids improve hormonal balance; and its protein-
bonded vitamins and minerals, as found in all whole
foods, assimilate better than the synthetic variety. Spirulina can generally be considered an appropriate food
for those who exercise vigorously, as evidenced by the
many world-class athletes who use it."[55]

These are some of the astounding health benefits of
chlorella and spirulina[56].

What can these two superfoods really do for your
health? They offer a stunning array of health benefits.
Chlorella and Spirulina have been shown to be effective
in treating and even reportedly <u>reversing</u> the following
conditions:

- Obesity

- Diabetes

- Hypoglycemia

- Severe liver damage and liver disorders

- High blood pressure

- Constipation

- Infections

- Inflammation of joints and tissues

- Body odor / breath odor

- Essential fatty acid deficiencies

- Mineral deficiencies (magnesium is a common deficiency)

Both Chlorella and Spirulina are particularly useful for:

- People with poor digestion and assimilation (these micro-algae are easy to digest and absorb)

- People with poor vitality and anemia

- Individuals who consumer large quantities of animal protein (the micro-algae protein, in contrast, is easier to digest and offers a far healthier balance of minerals)

- People who eat refined or processed foods

- People who take prescription drugs (Spirulina protects the kidneys and liver.)

- People who are overweight or obese

- People who engage in physical exercise and / or strength training

- People with low energy levels (feeling depleted, exhausted, etc.)

Resveratrol

I take one capsule every morning as part of the routine.

Did you know that resveratrol has cancer-fighting properties?

That the anti-aging benefits of resveratrol are so powerful that some have dubbed it the "Fountain of Youth"?

Resveratrol is an anti-inflammatory, increases energy levels, lowers blood sugar and extends life.

Resveratrol and anti-aging

It is believed that resveratrol works as an effective anti-aging ingredient. This is because resveratrol is thought to stimulate the SIRT-1 gene; SIRT-1, known as "the rescue gene", is the gene responsible for reducing fat stores during low-calorie diets. When the SIRT-1 gene is activated, it produces proteins that protect cells from inflammation and oxidative stress, two of the primary causes of premature aging and many degenerative diseases.

Stimulation of the SIRT-1 gene also seems to help slow down the aging process. Further study is needed, but many people swear by the anti-aging benefits of resveratrol in their diets. People looking for additional ways to slow down the aging process might try introducing this antioxidant to their health regimen as a way of enhancing it.

Dr. David Sinclair of Harvard is a leading researcher in the field of mitochondria and resveratrol. Dr. Sinclair's research has led him to believe that he potentially has found a key to extending our QOL and longevity by decades as reported in an article in the 2009 January issue of *Men's Health Magazine*. It involves the sirtuins, and specifically SIR2, which could be triggered by resveratrol. In 2008, Dr. Sinclair's Sirtris Pharmaceutical, a company he cofounded to develop anti-aging drugs, announced it had developed a chemical compound that was 1000 times more potent than resveratrol. In June of 2008, pharmaceutical powerhouse GlaxoSmithKline bought the company for $720 million; Sinclair believes that the sirtuin-activating, mitochondria-supercharged drug could be available in less than 10 years.

Resveratrol report on 60 Minutes

The buzz about resveratrol benefits reached a fever pitch when the antioxidant was featured on the news show "60 Minutes". Correspondent Morley Safer spoke with doctors and researchers regarding the various purported health benefits of resveratrol, bringing it to the attention of millions of television viewers around the world. Those who may have been reluctant to believe the hype surrounding this product were generally very impressed that a major show like "60 Minutes" would feature it so prominently.[57]

Vitamin B complex

I take one B-complex vitamin daily, and have for many years. This is one of the original vitamin supplements of which I have been a daily user. B-complex vitamins reportedly have many health benefits, including:

- Ease Stress

- Treat anxiety and depression

- Aid memory

- Relieve PMS

- Reduce heart-disease risk

The 11 members of what's known as the vitamin B complex are critical nutrients for all things mind-related; mood, memory, and even migraines can benefit from the Bs. In the right amounts, the Bs can quell anxiety, lift depression, ease PMS, and boost energy, and getting them couldn't be easier. The B vitamins are a chemically related family of nutrients that work as a team. Their mood-boosting and other health benefits (see chart below) result from intricate behind-the-scenes work in the body. Some B vitamins help cells burn fats and glucose for energy. Others help make neurotransmitters like serotonin. And some Bs assist with the production and repair of DNA. Many of us don't get enough Bs; according to the USDA, deficiencies in folic acid, B12, and B6 are especially common. Ensuring that your diet contains plenty of B-rich foods—dark-green vegetables, protein from animal sources, and whole grains—is critical. If your stress level is high or your mood feels off-kilter, or if your diet is low in Bs, you'll benefit from the higher amounts found in supplements.

Find the best B complex

To get the most benefits from any of the Bs, you need all of them, so start with a B-complex supplement that contains all 11. With the right B complex as a foundation, you can add larger amounts of individual Bs depending on your health concerns. The Bs are best taken with food—they can cause nausea when taken on an empty stomach—and early in the day. Vitamin B6 increases neurotransmitter activity; when taken late in the day, it can lead to increased dreaming, resulting in a restless night's sleep[58].

Osteo Bi-Flex

Glucosamine with MSM

Two tablets daily; these can be taken at separate times; however, I take both in the morning with everything else. I have read that it is much better to take the Osteo brand, as that supplement is the best absorbed. The trick to this is buying them on sale, because they are a tad on the expensive side. Again, in my opinion and why I take all of the mentioned supplements, they work for me, and I am a really active guy. Some of the benefits of Osteo Bi-Flex are:

- Doctor—recommended

- Helps renew cartilage & lubricate joints for joint comfort

- Promotes joint flexibility, comfort and range of motion by helping to support joint cartilage health over time.

- Glucosamine
  - *Glucosamine is a natural compound that is found in healthy cartilage.*
  - *Glucosamine sulfate is a normal constituent of glycoaminoglycans in the cartilage matrix and synovial fluid.*
  - *Available evidence from randomized controlled trials supports the use of glucosamine sulfate in*

the treatment of osteoarthritis, particularly of the knee.

- *Use of complementary therapies, including glucosamine, is common in patients with osteoarthritis, and may allow for reduced doses of non-steroidal anti-inflammatory agents[59].*

- Chondroitin

  - *Chondroitin sulfates increase the intrinsic viscosity of the synovial liquid.*

  - *Many literature data show that chondroitin sulfate could have an anti-inflammatory activity and a chondroprotective action by modifying the structure of cartilage.*

  - *Chondroitin provides cartilage with strength and resilience[60].*

"Roses are God's autograph of beauty, fragrance and love."

~Paul Bragg

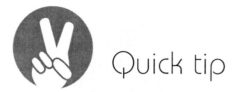

Quick tip

An estimated 21 million adults in the United States live with osteoarthritis--one of the most common types of arthritis. Osteoarthritis, also called degenerative joint disease, is caused by the breakdown of cartilage, which is the connective tissue that cushions the ends of bones within the joint. It is characterized by pain, joint damage, and limited motion. The disease generally occurs late in life, and most commonly affects the hands and large weight-bearing joints. Although the disease can impact several joints, the knees are often affected. Age, female gender, and obesity are risk factors for this condition[61].

Green Tea

I have developed a fondness for green tea in the brewed form (especially as an after dinner, pre-bedtime appetite killer). I do have the unenviable disease that afflicts so many of us – **later-night carbohydrate eats, or put it another way, "How to become a fat guy disease."** I was a Pop-tart, bowl of cereal, Oreo-loving night eater. Sneaking into the kitchen to grab a quickie made me eventually a 225 lb. chubster. A cup of green tea is a lifesaver, and brushing your teeth when you are getting the feeling of carbo eats disease works well also. And as another of my supplements, early morning in capsule form (500mg), green tea has its benefits, which reportedly include[62]:

- Protects against cancer.

- Aids in a weight-loss regimen.

- Helps prevent heart disease.

- It's believed to reduce total cholesterol, as well as LDL-cholesterol. This resulted in lower platelet aggregation, which then helps keep your blood pressure in check.

- Retards the aging process

- Green tea acts as an antiviral agent.

- The antioxidant levels of green tea are 100 times more effective than Vitamin C, and 25 times better than Vitamin E in protecting our immune systems.

- Calms digestion.

- Helps with bowel problems.

"Adopting a new healthier lifestyle can involve changing diet to include more fresh fruit and vegetables as well as increasing levels of exercise."

~Linford Christie

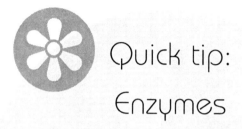

Quick tip:

Enzymes

The leaders in natural medicine refer to enzymes as "the li'l spark of life", because they turn what we eat into energy and are unlocking-mechanisms for energy use. Supplementation of your enzymes from a plant source is highly recommended. As you know, I highly recommend "Bragg Foods" and their "Braggzyme", which is an all-natural, vegan product[63].

Coenzyme Q10

CoQ10 (ubiquinone) has no known toxic side effects and has been the feature of numerous studies; I take one capsule (200mg) daily. The more I investigated this supplement the more I wondered what took me so long to start. It is a fat-soluble, vitamin-like substance that has been linked to energy production in cells, and is an antioxidant. Studies as far back as 1990 (*Journal of Clinical Pharmacology*) showed that 150mg of CoQ10 reduced angina attacks by upwards of 46 percent and increased physical performance. Coenzyme Q10 (or CoQ10) is a natural chemical compound that we make in our bodies and consume in our diets, primarily from oily fish, organ meats such as liver, and whole grains.

It resides in the energy-producing part of cells and is involved with producing a key molecule known as adenosine-5-triphosphate (or ATP). ATP is a cell's major energy source and it contributes to several important biological processes, such as the production of protein and muscle contraction.

Additional benefits of Coenzyme Q10 are:

- CoQ10 has the potential to vastly improve human health.

- It helps boost athletic performance (CoQ10 levels are low in people who exercise excessively.), and it improves exercise tolerance in people with muscular dystrophy.

- The American Chemical Society's most prestigious honor, the Priestley Medal, was awarded to Karl Folkers, Ph.D., for his landmark Coenzyme Q10 (CoQ10) research. That's because Folkers found that in addition to the benefits listed above, CoQ10's most valuable role may lie in fighting heart disease.

- CoQ10 levels tend to be lower in people with a high cholesterol count, compared with healthy individuals of the same age.

- What's more, certain cholesterol-lowering drugs (statins such as cerivastatin, atorvastatin, pravastatin, simvastatin and lovastatin) seem to reduce the natural levels of CoQ10 in the body.

- Taking CoQ10 supplements can correct the deficiency caused by statins, without changing the medication's positive effects on cholesterol levels.

- As a result of its beneficial effects on one of the body's most important organs, Folkers calls CoQ10 "a natural and essential co-factor in the heart."

- Of course, managing cholesterol levels, helping the circulatory system, blood sugar levels and heart health is particularly important for diabetics, and CoQ10 supplements may be a help to them.

- Despite concern that CoQ10 may cause a sudden drop in blood sugar, two recent studies of people with diabetes given CoQ10 twice a day showed they experienced no hypoglycemic response. If you're diabetic, *talk to your doctor about how you can safely take CoQ10.*

- Now, scientists are hoping its effects on the heart, blood systems, and tissue toxicity means CoQ10 can soon be used as part of a treatment program for Alzheimer's disease, and for recovery from stroke. They're also hopeful about the possibility of using it as part of a treatment regimen for women with breast cancer (together with conventional treatment and a nutritional program involving high levels of other antioxidants and fatty acids)[64].

> "Your waistline is your lifeline."
> ~Jack Lalanne

Aspirin

Acetylsalicylic acid was discovered by Arthur Eichengrun, a chemist with the German company Bayer. I found different dates for this discovery; suffice to say it was in the early 1800s. Aspirin, or acetylsalicylic acid, is a derivative of salicylic acid that is a mild, nonnarcotic analgesic useful in the relief of headache and muscle and joint aches. The drug works by inhibiting the production of prostaglandins, body chemicals that are necessary for blood clotting and which also sensitize nerve endings to pain.

This is one of the wonder drugs of our time; you know when you start to shop for aspirin (baby aspirin especially) and the price has gone through the roof, something must be up. I have come up with my own plan to combat the increase in the price of aspirin, which is this: buy the standard giant size generic bottle and break the tablets in half. The one-tablet dose is 325mg, and breaking it in half gives me about 164mg, just about the same size as two baby aspirin. You will save up to 50% in some big-box stores. One-half of a tablet in the morning does the trick for me. Aspirin has reportedly many positive attributes, including the potential to decreases the likelihood of blood clots forming in your blood vessels, which could trigger a heart attack or stroke[65].

Vitamin D

I know that the benefits of the "sunshine vitamin", Vitamin D, has been discussed ad nauseam lately, but the benefits are hard to discount. I will admit that living in the Midwest for most of my life (I did have those fifteen years in sunny Southern California in my younger, wilder days.), you tend to get that cabin fever light-deprivation feeling. And I will admit that I do use a tanning bed occasionally in the winter (I understand the health issues); however, it does seem to really help take the edge off, and now there is some evidence that it is clinically tested to help alleviate the winter blahs. My oral dosage to give me my adequate level is 2000 IU daily, again with my routine in the morning.

Vitamin D Benefits for Winter Weather Woes

Don't let the change in season shortchange you on Vitamin D benefits for mood, cold and flu resistance, and general health. Medical research suggests that upping the intake of Vitamin D may be one of the best ways to "winterize" the body. In winter, when skies are gray and sunny days are few and far between, getting plenty of the sunshine vitamin is more important than ever. Keeping levels of the vitamin high during the winter months is particularly important for people over 60, since the body's ability to manufacture Vitamin D declines with age.

Do you need more vitamin D?

Chances are the answer is yes, particularly if you're over 50.

Initially recognized mainly for its importance to healthy bones, Vitamin D has recently been identified as crucial to virtually all aspects of health, from preventing cardiovascular disease and perhaps even certain types of cancer to helping with mood management and even improving urinary incontinence. At the same time, Vitamin D deficiency has been identified as a worldwide problem. Low levels of the vitamin have been associated with a number of serious diseases including cardiovascular disease, multiple sclerosis, asthma, Alzheimer's disease, and several forms of cancer.

Recent research has also shown that insufficient levels of the vitamin are clearly correlated with mental health issues, including depression and cognitive impairment in the elderly[66].

45: Sample day from the body-building show

What I like to call my "hand food" is just an easy way to describe the daily routine that I have developed thanks to the BB show. Here is an example of my food journal during the show, which is remarkably similar, almost exactly the same, as today:

This was taken from March 5, 2010

- 4:30 am- Homemade juice, 1ice cube of wheat grass in water, 1 tablespoon of Nutiva coconut oil, 1 tablespoon of Carlson's Fish Oil, daily vitamin supplement routine mentioned earlier, Bragg's apple cider vinegar (1-oz) with water and cinnamon

- 7:30 am- Post-workout shake (1 scoop hemp protein, 1 scoop whey protein, ½ scoop L-Glutamine, 2 tablespoons of steel-cut oats)

- 9:00 am- Small bowl of steel-cut oat cereal with water, ½ cup raisins, 3-4 prunes, ¼ teaspoon of cinnamon

- 11:00 am- 1 banana, 1 whole lemon, 1 whole apple

- 11:30 am- Homemade granola (small handful of almonds, small handful of whole pumpkin seeds, 3 figs, 4 dates)

- 1:00 pm- Post-workout shake (same as 7:30 am)

- 3:00 pm- ½ sweet potato, 1 small piece of roast beef, 1 broccoli stalk (yes, the stalk) 1 lemon

- 5:00 pm- 1 tablespoon of coconut oil, 1 tablespoon Carlson's Fish Oil, 2 figs

- 7:30 pm- Small green salad and a piece of pork loin (Dinner)

- 9:00 pm- Air-popped popcorn (large bowl), glass of milk

- Of course water consumption is a given; I always drink at least 3 liters a day even during normal time. The rule of thumb is ½ your body weight in ounces per day.

As you can see, this looks like a lot of food. It actually equated to fewer than 2,000 calories for the day. With the double-session workouts, I was running about a 500 to 1,000 calorie deficit a day, which, over the 16 weeks, put me exactly where I needed to be weight-wise. After a while, you find what you like (it changes slightly from day to day), but the timing is always very similar. It is the pattern (call it habit; call it brain mapping; call it saving money; not eating out or eating junk)—I had no place for it in my day, none!

The key to all of this was the preparing of everything the night before, which is the ticket to success, and, again, where effort and planning are critical. To this day, I still am on a very similar routine, making daily food the night before, as soon as I get home, to have this out of my hair.

Understand that it is a major team effort; Sandy had everything in big bags in the fridge, and so, once a week or so, you need to have your prep stuff in mind. Don't think this happens by magic; it takes effort and planning. The absolute key is the knowing how, the experience, and the time-management skills

I think it is pretty self-explanatory when I mention hand food, but if it isn't, then here you go:

Hand food eating is anything you can eat right out of your lunch box without microwaving or using a utensil. Think of it as cave man eating; it's fast and easy. It will be your during-work food, and it completely eliminates any need to buy a candy bar, or eat a donut. Now we call all of this our "HyMEP".

Now that the show is over, I still maintain the mind-set of the schedule.

46: The everyday HyMEP

So, obviously you cannot stay in body-building prep mode forever. I mean, three percent body fat is impossible to maintain (and not healthy), for the long term. So what is the daily routine?

Remember, I talked about the "hand food", and "timing" and "prep", and the most obvious thing to me about doing the prep for the show was how good I felt, that I shaved down about 18 pounds in 16 weeks and frankly felt pretty good. The routine is the key that I want to emphasize; it is the backbone of our HyMEP.

Timing is everything, balance is key, and quality is important.

Here is a regular day for me, types of foods and timing. Please use this as a reference and a guide, ease into it, and remember it is only a framework and getting your nutrition under control is a process.

- Of course we pack our daily food when I get home from work; that puts this out of the way for the next work day. I cannot emphasize enough how incredibly important this has become to my routine. Setting up your meal pattern for the next day not only gives you time in the morning; it also sets up the quality and type of snacks you need throughout the day. In addition, the money you save not buying impulse food will amaze you.

- Remember I have shared earlier the "Breakfast Routine" (juice, supplements, oils and water), early morning after your stretching.

- The following is an average meal day and the times that I eat (you see it's the timing and routine).

- Apples, 2—I always try and eat one at 9:00 am (plus the figs, prunes and sometimes a small handful of raisins, and dates from my granola—see below) and the other somewhere in the afternoon.

- Greek yogurt, 2 plain

- In a normal day I eat one of these after I work out at lunch time, since I do not make protein shakes every day, and the other as close to 3:00 as possible. The 3:00 pm yogurt is an unbelievable boost, rocket fuel!

- I do mix my homemade granola in my yogurt.

- Water.

- Homemade granola—basically what my friends call bird food. The fruit part of the granola is eaten with my first apple, around 9:00 am (I have read that an apple is much more of a stimulant in the morning than a cup of coffee), the nuts are mixed into your yogurt later in the day, for healthy fats and protein. The recipe for the granola is as follows:

- 1 small handful of almonds

- 1 small handful of raw pumpkin seeds

- 3-4 dried figs

- 3-4 dried dates (Sandy's favorite, and these have helped her tremendously with sweet tooth cravings)

- 3-4 prunes

- Sandwich bag of mixed vegetables, considered complex carbohydrates and full of fiber (these can be eaten at any time you wish throughout the day; they are free calories), including but not limited to:

  - *Broccoli—which is high in fiber and has been shown to have cholesterol-lowering benefits, is rich in sulfur compounds, which are good for the liver and thus strengthen our natural filtration and detoxification systems.*

  - *Baby carrots—improve vision, cancer prevention, anti-aging, can help prevent stroke according to Harvard research, prevent heart disease and are high in fiber*

  - *Celery—lowers blood pressure, heart disease risk and cholesterol, plus has natural chemi-*

cals to fight cancer. High in fiber and is consid-ered a negative calorie.

- *Radishes—low calorie, high fiber, loaded with Vitamin C, and another cancer fighter.*

- Water.

- Banana—which is a great compliment to the noonish Greek yogurt, and has two times as many carbohydrates as an apple, five times as much Vitamin A and iron and three times as much phosphorus. In addition, bananas are also rich in potassium and natural sugars. All of these factors combined make the banana a "superfood" that is an integral part of a healthy daily regimen.

- Water

- Lemon—I know what people are going to say; I hear it all the time. LEMON? Yes, I eat a lemon a day, peeled like an orange, in the late morn-ing. It is refreshing and helps keep that pH level even. Once you get used to the taste, they are frankly outstanding. Health benefits of lemons that have been known for centuries. The two biggest are lemons' strong antibacterial, anti-viral, and immune-boosting powers and their use as a weight-loss aid because lemon juice is a digestive aid and liver cleanser. Lemons contain many substances--notably citric acid, calcium, magnesium, Vitamin C, bioflavonoids, pectin, and limonene--that promote immunity and fight infection.

- Water

- If we have any leftover meat from dinner (chicken, beef, and fish) I cut it into small hand-sized pieces and put it into sandwich bags. One of these baggies is a great addition to your afternoon snack, but I do not have meat every day.

- Water

So there you go, a road map, a starting point, something to consider. I do not expect anyone to copy my routine; the point of sharing this is that it works, it is sustainable, and you will feel great.

Having done your prep the day before keeps those early morning issues from screwing with your daily food. Because, as you can see this is not lunch, and the three-meal-a-day mindset needs to go away. New conditioning, slowly, can start to make a big difference in you QOL, your energy, and your happiness.

After work—5:00

Here is the post-work routine; yes, unless I have a workout session after work, it's time to quell the hungries.

- Homemade glass of juice with a scoop of hemp protein, 6-oz. glass

- One oz. of Bragg's Apple Cider Vinegar, same glass, with water and sprinkle of cinnamon

- One tablespoon of Nutiva Organic coconut oil

- One tablespoon of Carlson's Fish Oil

Now we make the food supply for tomorrow; get it done now, because I have to do a talk show in like less than an hour and I need to prep. And I know Mr. Procrastinator (me), will not get things done otherwise, so it's all about the routine, so throw it together. Remember I talked about the hand food; well, it is helpful in two ways. First it is easy and fast to eat, and secondly it is easy and fast to put together, as long as you have your plan.

It should be around 5:20, and now I make a cup of green tea, a cup of coffee, and a bottle of water (sounds like a lot), and head upstairs to the studio to prep for the radio show, which we do three times a week (as of right now anyway); at some point we will go to five days.

Radio talk show from 5:40ish, on air from 6:00 until 7:00 and then follow-up calls, until around 7:15ish.

We try and have a light dinner around 7:30, Sandy is a doll and team player, and will normally have something ready. Remember one of the key ingredients to the HyMEP is that family socialization. We are not yet quite completely empty-nesters (we are half way there), but maybe some of you boomers are; make a point to catch up at the table—it is very important to share your day with your family.

Dinner

If it is show night (M-W-F) we sit together at around 7:15 and have a somewhat light dinner. Always salad, with a main course, and we do a lot of quinoa, sweet potato, brown rice types of carbs. This meal is kind of a freebie; you really should not be all that hungry, so just eat a little bit slower, and the socialization is really big. Now I know that they say you should not watch television while you eat; however, we catch up on the news, and often share our day and comment together on current events. The HyMEP, like the traditional Mediterranean, involves that socialization; it really is a huge blessing and component to maintaining that homeostasis.

On non-show nights it is not unusual to have our "fend for yourself" night; normally there are plenty of choices. Sometimes we will do our traditional, other times fend, but again it is not that big of a deal because we have built a good day around mindful eating.

Snack

Invariably an 8 to 9 pm snack is needed to quiet the rumblings every night, and we may need to adjust our dinner menu; a few times a week is no big deal, it just has to be a quality snack, and watch the portion sizes. My air-popped popcorn bowl is Jethro-sized, really, but because it is air popped, with coconut oil and sea salt, it sure beats the heck out of sugary cereal, or my dreaded Pop-tarts (those things made me fat), cookies or something else that is on the no-way list. So Jethro bowl or not, it works.

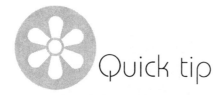

Quick tip

Sugary snacks will make you hungrier, and lead you to eat more of the same because of the blood sugar spike, so watch it!

An almond milk protein shake is a great snack; use a scoop of whey protein, ½ glass (4 ounces) of almond or skim milk with water, sprinkle a small amount of cinnamon and there you go.

Green tea is another winner in my world, as is something as simple as brushing my teeth. It's amazing how that will knock the hungries right down.

Guaranteed Results Tips for Eating

1. Water consumption is by far the top tip on my list; we all need to increase our daily consumption to equal approximately ½ our body weight in ounces. So for example, a 200-pound person should consume 100 ounces throughout their day. Whole chapters and books have been written on this topic, but let's keep it simple and just get it done; you will be amazed by the way you feel.

2. Limit or eliminate high fructose soft drinks, alcohol, sugary beverages and all energy drinks.

3. Eliminate partially hydrogenated oils (trans fat) and prepared packaged foods.

4. Eat as many whole food/one item foods as possible. Examples of such foods are fruits (apples, oranges), vegetables, raw or steamed (broccoli, celery, carrots), chicken, eggs, beef, nuts and seeds.

5. Understand the importance of maintaining an even PH level in your body, and how important it is to healthy and practicable weight management. PH level is critical to the correct absorption of vitamins and minerals.

6. Learn to incorporate eating small meals/snacks throughout your day, preferably six (for example every three hours), spaced out evenly to keep your metabolism running on high and keeping your energy level high.

7. Never skip breakfast.

8. Try not to eat two hours prior to your bedtime.

9. Understand the ratio of macronutrients and their consumption. 20-30% proteins, 20-30% fats, 40-60% carbohydrates.

10. Utilize a multi-vitamin along with good quality liquid fish oil, flax meal, and other healthy fat sources.

11. Balance; try and consume a wide variety of foods from different sources.

12. Small steps are the key—Think about this, if you eliminate just 200 calories a day (for example one soda), and increase your movement (two 10-minute sessions of something), a 400-calorie shift daily, you could potentially lose 20 pounds in one year!

47: The Chemicals within us

Understanding the synergistic qualities of our cardiovascular system, brain health, and therefore QOL lead us to how movement can increase vital chemicals within our bodies. I have listed some of the key neurotransmitters and hormones that play an important role in our longevity, health, happiness and QOL. Many studies have proven that movement and exercise play a critical role in this aspect of our lives. It is very important to all of us boomers to have a solid grasp of these compounds, as it relates to fitness and aging.

Hormones, which play a critical role in our bodies, are chemical messengers secreted from glands to cells within tissues or organs in the body. They also maintain chemical levels in the bloodstream to help achieve homeostasis, which contributes to our state of balance within the body.

Hormones transport information and directions from one group of cells to another. In the human body, hormones influence almost every cell, organ and function. They control our growth, development, metabolism, tissue function, sexual function, reproduction, the way our bodies use food, the response of our bodies to emergencies and even our moods.

The following are some of the key hormones and chemicals within us.

BDNF

Brain-derived neurotrophic factor is the name of a protein released when you exercise. It boosts the function and growth of neurons (remember neurogenesis). BDNF is like a glue; it binds receptors at your synapses (nerves), which unleashes a flow of ions to increase voltage and increase signal strength. As always we have to think about the electrical and chemical nature of our bodies, signals, networks and receptors, which in turn activate genes, which cause the call for production of more BDNF.

Dr. John Ratey, in his book called *Spark: The Revolutionary New Science of Exercise and the Brain* (*"Spark: The Revolutionary New Science of Exercise and the Brain"*, *Dr. John Ratey, Little Brown, 2008*), calls BDNF "Miracle-Gro for the Brain". This is good, because BDNF just isn't a very catchy name, whereas Miracle-Gro is at least something you've heard of, but bottom line is: exercise intensifies your amount of Miracle-Gro, makes your brain better at growing the connections (think farmer and planting seeds), and routes (myelin), that help you learn and remember and be smarter and more knowledgeable.

A study in the journal *Medicine and Science in Sports and Exercise*[67] found that levels of BDNF increased 13 percent after just 30 minutes of high-intensity exercise, but showed no increase after low-intensity exercise. The bottom line is this: try for two high-intensity sessions a week, or mix in HIIT training throughout your workout to achieve your 30 minutes.

Regular physical exercise stimulates the central nervous system, which increases the transport of oxygen to the brain as well as cerebral metabolic activity of various neurotransmitters, including dopamine, serotonin, norepinephrine, and acetylcholine.

The efficacy of exercise to reduce stress and improve mental well-being is well-founded and supported; it is hypothesized that exercise "detoxifies", or gets rid of the stress-related hormones quickly. This could be a result of the increased metabolism from exercise.

In addition to the countless physical benefits, exercise can have psychological benefits. Studies show that exercise can increase the amounts of the neurotransmitters dopamine and serotonin in your brain. The increased levels of neurotransmitters can help treat disorders such as Parkinson's disease and depression, as well as help you to feel more energetic overall.

Your brain produces the neurotransmitters serotonin and dopamine so that your brain cells can communicate. According to McGill University's website, dopamine helps your brain execute motor movements and regulate your mood and concentration. Your brain uses serotonin to regulate your body temperature, mood, and appetite, among other things. Low levels of serotonin are thought to cause depression.

Dopamine

Dopamine is a neurotransmitter that helps control the brain's reward and pleasure centers. Dopamine, a stimulant, makes people more talkative and excitable, and affects brain processes that control movement, emotional response, and ability to experience pleasure and pain. Dopamine also helps regulate movement and emotional responses, and it enables us not only to see rewards, but to take action to move toward them. It increases saliency, the ability to focus, giving us the ability to see something when it stands out.

Dopamine deficiency results in Parkinson's disease, and people with low dopamine activity may be more prone to addiction. The presence of a certain kind of dopamine receptor is also associated with sensation-seeking. Its main function as a hormone is to inhibit the release of prolactin from the anterior lobe of the pituitary.

An important neurotransmitter (messenger) in the brain, dopamine is a precursor (forerunner) of adrenaline[68].

Exercise and Dopamine

In a May 2007 article in the *Journal of Neuroscience*, neuroscientist Gizelle Petzinger and colleagues note that exercise may cause the brain cells that use dopamine to work more efficiently. The study shows that the dopamine-releasing neurons of rats that ran on a treadmill released more dopamine than rats that did not exercise. The dopamine also remained active longer in the rats that ran on a treadmill.

Exercise may help people who suffer from Parkinson's disease by reducing damage to brain cells that release dopamine. In an August 2007 article in the journal *Neuroscience Letters*, M. C. Yoon and colleagues reported that rats that exercised on a treadmill 30 minutes a day for two weeks lost less dopamine-releasing cells than rats that performed no exercise.

Serotonin

Serotonin is a chemical (neurotransmitter) that helps maintain a "happy feeling" and seems to help keep our moods under control by helping with sleep, calming anxiety, and relieving depression. Serotonin acts both as a chemical messenger that transmits nerve signals between nerve cells, and that causes blood vessels to narrow.

In addition to being involved in the process of addiction, low serotonin levels are believed to be the reason for many cases of mild to moderate depression, which can lead to symptoms like anxiety, apathy, fear, feelings of worthlessness, insomnia and fatigue. We are learning that depression is related to a number of other health issues.

Depression is the nation's most prevalent mental health problem, affecting about 15 million Americans who spend about $3 billion a year on drugs to battle it. Almost all of these medicines target either serotonin or norepinephrine, brain chemicals that are neurotransmitters.

Exercise and Serotonin

In a November 2007 article in the *Journal of Psychiatry & Neuroscience*, Dr. Simon Young notes that exercise may increase the amount of serotonin in your brain, referencing studies that indicate that physical activity results in higher levels of the molecules 5-HIAA and tryptophan in the body. The body uses 5-HIAA and tryptophan to produce serotonin.

Benefits of Increased Serotonin

In that same article, Dr. Simon Young notes that exercise is commonly used as a treatment for mild depression, because of its serotonin-increasing effects. Dr. Young says that aerobic exercise, such as jogging, biking and swimming, works best to treat mild depression. Also, according to *Fitness Magazine*, the increase in serotonin from aerobic exercise boosts your energy levels[69] [and[70]].

Norepinephrine

Norepinephrine (adrenalin) is considered a neurotransmitter and a hormone and has many important functions. As a stress hormone, norepinephrine affects portions of the brain, such as the amygdala, the part of the limbic system where its primary role is memory and emotional reactions. This is where attention responses are controlled. Norepinephrine works alongside epinephrine and adrenaline to give the body sudden energy in times of stress, known as the "fight or flight" response. As a neurotransmitter, it passes nerve impulses from one neuron to the next.

Doctors use norepinephrine to help regulate blood conditions or use medication to increase levels of the neurotransmitter to alter brain chemistry and improve moods for patients with mental disorders.

Certain antidepressant medications increase levels of norepinephrine and serotonin, which are classified and described by physicians as "reuptake inhibitors" or

SNRIs. These drugs increase levels of serotonin and norepinephrine in patients suffering from depression, according to MayoClinic.com.

At the first sign of stress norepinephrine will tell the body to stop producing insulin. This gives the body plenty of fast-acting blood glucose (sugar), to activate energy stores. Norepinephrine, which restricts blood vessels and causes an increase in blood pressure, is a product of your adrenal gland system and is associated with the "stress hormone" cortisol[71].

Cortisol

I like to use the analogy with cortisol as our "cave man" mentality hormone; it is our ancient fear of starving, or being eaten by a Saber-toothed tiger, that makes cortisol so powerful; it is our "stress hormone".

The body resists weight loss if it is exposed to stress for a long time and the cortisol level stays high. The body thinks it is hard times and that it is hungry. Therefore it holds on to all the foods consumed and the fat already stored in the body. Research has shown that sustained stress can damage the hippocampus, the part of the limbic brain central to learning and memory. The culprits are "glucocorticoids", a class of steroid hormones secreted from the adrenal glands during stress. They are more commonly known as corticosteroids or cortisol. Recall the term "homeostasis", the balance of everything within us; hormones and neurotransmitters are some of the key elements that must stay in balance. Without homeostasis trouble is brewing in River City.

Cortisol is a catabolic hormone, and as such it tells the body what protein, fat, or carbohydrates to burn depending on what challenge the body faces. Cortisol is also the hormone that tells your body that the stress is gone and to stop making the stimulants adrenalin, norepinephrine and epinephrine. It is a major player in the creation of belly fat, and therefore carries the tag of "bad hormone". This is a misnomer, because as with anything and everything, balance and moderation is the key—same with Cortisol. As the principal long-acting stress hormone that assists in the body's ability to mobilize fuel, cue up attention and memory, recall T-Rex chasing our ancestors and eating them, cortisol prepares our body for the chase.

Cortisol influences blood sugar, especially on how the body uses fuel. Cortisol also has the clout to both take the fat in the form of triglycerides and move it to the muscle (a very good thing), or break down muscle and convert it into glycogen for more energy (at times a very bad thing). In addition, cortisol will increase cravings for high-fat and high-carb foods, lower the leptin levels and stimulate your appetite. Remember leptin is a mediator of long-term regulation of energy balance, suppressing food intake and thereby inducing weight loss, so in essence cortisol blocks our ability to lose the extra pounds. If stress is present, cortisol is automatically put into action.

Cortisol is an important hormone with dual faces. Information shows that under stress cortisol "greases" nerves to assist in their elasticity and adaptability, so that stress can be tolerated and managed. This data is consistent with the release of BDNF (brain-derived neurotropic factor) under stress, which also maintains plasticity while helping nerves form new connections. A picture of synergy emerges as to how nerves tolerate stress and successfully overcome challenges, even adapting to new forms of ongoing stress. This requires adequate cortisol and BDNF working together—homeostasis and balance, which is teamwork at its finest. If cortisol runs low then nerves overheat. If BDNF runs low then nerves die and new changes cannot be made. Stress is a good thing, in certain circumstances; we need stress to stay sharp, and it keeps us on our game. However, it is that always-present stress that starts to throw the balance out of whack, and therein lies the problem.

Chronic over-secretion of stress hormones adversely affects brain function, especially memory. Too much cortisol can prevent the brain from laying down a new memory, or from accessing already-existing memories. At high or inexorable concentrations cortisol can have a toxic effect on neurons, which can erode the contacts (think operator patching through a phone call that falls asleep, so the call does not go through); we need to keep the operator happy and alert.

During a perceived threat, the adrenal glands immediately release adrenalin. If the threat is severe or still persists after a couple of minutes, the adrenals then release cortisol. Once in the brain, cortisol remains much longer than adrenalin, where it continues to affect brain cells.

Cortisol and memory

Have you ever forgotten something during a stressful situation that you should have remembered? Cortisol also interferes with the function of our neurotransmitters, the compounds that brain cells use to communicate with each other. Excessive cortisol can make it difficult to think or retrieve long-term memories. That's why people get confused and jumbled in a severe crisis. Their mind goes blank because "the lines are down." They can't remember where the fire exit is, for example.

Stress hormones divert blood glucose to exercising muscles; therefore the amount of glucose – hence energy – that reaches the brain's hippocampus is diminished. This creates an energy crisis in the hippocampus, which compromises its ability to create new memories. That may be why some people can't remember a very traumatic event, and why short-term memory is usually the first casualty of age-related memory loss resulting from a lifetime of stress.

Normally, in response to stress, the brain's hypothalamus secretes a hormone that causes the pituitary gland to secrete another hormone that causes the adrenals to secrete cortisol. When levels of cortisol rise to a certain level, several areas of the brain – especially the hippocampus – tell the hypothalamus to turn off the cortisol-producing mechanism; this is the proper feedback response.

Because the hippocampus is part of the feedback mechanism that signals when to stop cortisol production, a damaged hippocampus causes cortisol levels to get out of control – further compromising memory and cognitive function. The cycle of degeneration then continues (similarly to the deterioration of the pancreas-insulin feedback system).

Acetylcholine

...is a neurotransmitter, which means it helps the nerves to communicate, and it is important for our entire network of nerves in our central nervous system to communicate; it is the "link" between muscles and our nervous system. Acetylcholine is needed in all individuals to have healthy signals between nerve cells in the brain that also move out to the larger skeletal muscles.

Acetylcholine is found in egg yolks and helps keep our memories sharp. Acetylcholine is also necessary for learning and to preserve short-term memory.

When acetylcholine is released at a neuromuscular junction, the area of contact between the ends of a large "myelinated nerve fiber" and a fiber of skeletal muscle, acetylcholine crosses the tiny space (synapse) that separates the nerve from the muscle. It then binds to the receptor molecules on the muscle fiber's surface. This initiates a chain of events that lead to muscle contraction.

To understand the importance of acetylcholine, consider that its deficiency can result in the inability to contract larger muscles and the heart ceasing to beat; also low levels of acetylcholine have been noted in Alzheimer's disease.

Certain B vitamins are critical for the synthesis of acetylcholine, and a deficiency in them can cause decreased acetylcholine production. These include vitamin B1, B5 and B12, which are available as supplements. Also, the herb ginkgo biloba reportedly stimulates the brain's absorption of acetylcholine, and the lipid phosphatidylserine, which aids in the production and release of acetylcholine into the brain.

Endorphins

Long known to occur after intense exercise, some refer to endorphins, hormones produced in your body, as releasing the "runner's high"; they are a very powerful natural painkiller, which have been linked to that all-day feel-good often accompanied by a positive and energizing outlook on life.

They are related to opiates, and give us the peaceful mellow bliss, satisfaction and pleasure. A narcotic-like substance that can block pain, endorphin is one of the body's own painkillers, an opioid (morphine-like) chemical produced by the body. Endorphins act as analgesics (pain relievers), and are released by certain neurotransmitters.

One of the major benefits of endorphins is they are noted not to be as addictive as morphine, although they generate the same feeling of delight.

Reportedly endorphins may actually improve your body's insulin action, thereby reversing or reducing insulin resistance.

Testosterone

A naturally occurring androgenic (male) hormone, testosterone encourages growth of bone (Wolff's law), and muscle. It helps maintain muscle strength in men, and has been used in treatments in small doses for women, relieving symptoms in some forms of metastatic breast cancer.

Testosterone is a hormone accountable for sex drive in both men and women.

Low testosterone levels have been linked to depression and low libido, memory problems and reportedly linked to Alzheimer's.

Low levels of this hormone in men have been linked to talk about male menopause, contributing to mid-life crisis and divorce. In addition, low levels of testosterone in women can affect sexuality and self-worth.

It should be noted that natural testosterone creation (grow our own) is the best way to counter act low levels. These include:

- Compound exercises—Multi-muscle group exercises, squats, rows, and bench presses are better for boosting testosterone levels than isolation moves, for example curls or triceps pushdowns.

- Do heavier sets—Find your 85 percent max (a weight you can only lift five times), and blow it up. Heavier, more powerful exertion lifts are more effective than high-rep, low-weight work.

- DO NOT OVERTRAIN—Recovery time is critical, as is sleep, seven to eight hours nightly. Over-training could cause testosterone levels to plunge by 40 percent according to a study conducted by the University of North Carolina. Never train the same muscle group two days in a row.

- Lose the beer belly—Being 30 percent or more overweight could raise a man's estrogen level, which leads to lower testosterone levels.

- Lose the weight slowly—Crash diets or cutting your calorie intake by more than 15 percent makes your brain think you're starving, so it shuts down testosterone production to wait out the deprivation. Starvation diets also promote cortisol levels to rise, which will increase fat storage and belly fat.

- Forget low carb diets, for example "Adkins". Studies suggests that eating a high-protein, low-carbohydrate diet can lower your testosterone levels. Your protein intake should be only around 16 percent of your daily calories. So, if you're the average 170-pound man who eats 2,900 calories a day, you should eat about 140 grams of protein daily, which is about the amount in two chicken breasts and a 6-ounce can of tuna.

- Grab your partner for morning sex—German scientists found that simply having an erection causes your testosterone to rise considerably, and puts a smile on both of your faces!

Oxytocin

Oxytocin is sometimes referred to as the "love hormone"; is a neuromodulator—in other words it *enhances* the overall effectiveness of synaptic change. It is a behavior and a game changer; large-scale brain reorganization occurs, and long-lasting effectiveness is enhanced. A lifetime of love possibility is enabled—remember "neuroplasticity"—brain remapping occurs.

Oxytocin, a natural chemical in the body that flows before and during climax, gets some of the credit for pleasure, along with a couple of other compounds like endorphins; orgasm is a powerful painkiller.

Tender feelings of warmth occur; trust and calm moods take effect.

Frequent and powerful orgasms increase the level of the orgasm hormone, oxytocin. The oxytocin level is linked to the personality, passion, social skills and emotional quotient (EQ), all of which affects career, marriage, emotions and social life. Orgasms are very beneficial for sexual health because they empower our pituitary (brain function).

Benefits of Oxytocin

Relationships require a lot of work and many times people think that communicating with a partner on stressful issues, like finances for instance, is not a possible thing to achieve. However, recent studies now show that oxytocin, also known as the "love hormone" could actually help to eradicate such conflicts in a relationship. In addition to being the "love hormone" oxytocin is responsible for:

Reducing anxiety—Oxytocin spray is also beneficial in times of anxiety or heightened fear. Oxytocin and biomedical therapies have proven to help diagnose autism-spectrum disorders in children. It also has an influence on insulin and glucagon, which regulate blood sugar levels in diabetic patients.

Improves sexual intimacy—A hug causes the release of oxytocin, leading to sexual intimacy, and even induces closeness between strangers. In fact, oxytocin plays a huge role in building relationships, promoting lasting relationships, strengthening marriages and even building warmth among strangers.

Relieves stress—Oxytocin deters the release of hormones responsible for stress known as cortisol, and also reduces blood pressure that occurs due to anxiety. It makes one feel relaxed, calm, affectionate, generous, trusting and calm. Additionally, it also improves sociability and reduces the feeling of isolation.

Estrogen

A hormone that comprises a group of mixtures, including estrone, estradiol and estriol, is the main sex hormone in women and is essential to the menstrual cycle. Although estrogen exists in men as well as women, it is found in higher amounts in women, especially those capable of reproducing.

Estrogen overload is a serious problem in aging men. One report showed that estrogen levels of the average 54-year-old man are higher than those of the average 59-year-old woman. This relates to our earlier talk about testosterone, as excess estrogen can cause the balance between the two to shift, which can induce some of the symptoms of lower testosterone.

Estrogen is an essential hormone for men, but too much causes a wide range of health problems. High serum levels of estrogen also fake the brain into thinking that enough testosterone is being created, thereby slowing the natural formation of testosterone. Estrogen loss in women due to pre-menopause and menopause is of serious concern; one major issue is osteoporosis.

Osteoporosis is a loss of bone mass that can begin any time after the age of 30. Bone, at its peak, is being broken down and built back up again on a regular basis (Wolff's law). When the bone being broken down is no longer being replaced to its fullest extent, bones lose density and can become fragile, and may be easily broken.

Reportedly most women who have reached menopause may be susceptible to bone loss, especially if they are not using hormone replacement therapy (HRT), which includes estrogen.

Baby boomer women, who engage in regular physical activity, for example walking, jogging or swimming, can alleviate some of the issues of bone loss associated with osteoporosis. I encourage women to practice weight training, utilizing free weights, machines or resistance bands, all of which put stress on your bones, which protects and increases your bone density.

Any household item that has any weight can be used as a weight-training tool; be creative—use a can of corn, a small sack of potatoes – anything, and practice, for example, with a compound move such as an overhead shoulder push while doing a squat. The more active you are, the better your bones will like it.

And really, ladies, we men need you around to tell us what to do! We have a bright future, we've paid our dues, and it's time to enjoy the "Indian summer" of our lives.

Melatonin

Melatonin is an important hormone that is made in our brains and is responsible for regulating other hormones, and more importantly melatonin regulates the body's sleep cycle. Very small quantities of it are found in foods such as meats, grains, fruits, and vegetables. You can also buy it as a supplement.

Melatonin is a strong antioxidant, and some evidence suggests it may support the immune cycle.

Certain studies have shown that melatonin improves depression and anxiety of post-menopausal women, and other studies have shown that some persons with depression and panic disorder have exhibited low levels of melatonin.

Melatonin is involved in female hormone production and does influence the menstrual cycle.

Melatonin has shown to have strong neuroprotective effects, both as an antioxidant and plaque preventer in the brain, which has been associated with reduced risk of Alzheimer's disease.

Since melatonin levels are highest when we are young, and diminish as we age, it is important to understand the benefits of supplemental use; it is safe and non-addictive, and is an excellent sleep aid. Dosages should be low and always consult a physician before use.

Scientists are also studying other uses for melatonin, such as:

- Treating seasonal affective disorder (SAD) due to light deprivation in winter months.

- Helping to regulate sleep patterns for individuals who work varying shifts.

- Preventing or reducing problems with sleeping and confusion after surgery.

- Reducing chronic cluster headaches.

Melatonin can have side effects, but these will subside once you stop taking the supplement. Side effects may include:

- Sleepiness

- Lower body temperature

- Vivid dreams

- Morning grogginess

- Small changes in blood pressure[72]

DHEA

Dehydroepiandrosterone (DHEA) is an androgen (male sex hormone) that is produced by both the adrenal glands and the ovaries. It is one of the most abundant hormones in the body, and if low levels exist in your body it can lead to adrenal fatigue.

DHEA has been reported to improve the ability to recover from episodes of stress and trauma, overwork, temperature extremes, etc. If a woman is suffering a decline in libido due to dwindling testosterone levels, often it is diminishing DHEA levels that are at the root of the testosterone deficiency, as DHEA is the main component the body uses to create testosterone.

DHEA also helps to protect and increase bone density, guards cardiovascular health by keeping "bad" cholesterol (LDL) levels under control, provides vitality and energy, sharpens the mind, and helps maintain normal sleep patterns.

For women, if the amount and occurrence of the stresses in your life—either those within (such as your perceptions about your life), or those external (such as having surgery or working the night shift)—become too great, then over time your adrenal glands will begin to become exhausted. This will mean that you are much more likely to suffer from fatigue and menopausal symptoms. A woman in a state of adrenal exhaustion is likely to find herself at a distinct disadvantage when entering perimenopause, because perimenopause itself is an additional form of stress.

Adrenal fatigue can be a terrible nemesis, and should be understood and addressed. Thyroid disorders can cause an energy breakdown, which could lead to over-working of your adrenal glands and eventual exhaustion. Although supplemental forms of DHEA are available, I would encourage a more holistic approach with lifestyle changes including:

- Focus more on loving thoughts

- Allow yourself to accept nurturing and affection: Daily affirmations (I use Facebook) to start your day off on a positive note work well. Write a quick note to someone you care about, share good feelings; write these in the early morning to get your mind pointed in the right direction.

- Follow a healthy, whole foods diet with minimal sugar and adequate protein: Excessive sugar intake in our diets is ruining our consistent energy patterns and causing issues with inflammation.

- Multivitamins and supplements work well: Refer back to the section on HyMEP (hybrid Mediterranean eating plan), and healthy fats. Energy levels and mitochondrial efficiencies depend on a level, evenly paced diet.

- Adequate sleep: Maintaining 7 to 9 hours of sleep has been shown to combat adrenal fatigue.

- Very light movement/exercise: Overdoing your exercise can put additional stress on your adrenals, which can cause fatigue; walking is a great movement for combatting fatigue.

- Natural sunlight has been indicated as a treatment, but be careful not to overexpose yourself. Vitamin D supplementation has been used and reportedly is effective.

- Finally quit over-committing: In our hectic 21st century world we try and do too much; slow down, do what you can, and learn to say NO! We must become more accountable for our own health; in essence that is why I wrote this book in the first place, to improve accountability to ourselves. Doing for others all of the time will eventually wear you out; everyone needs their own special time for themselves, so relax and give to yourself.

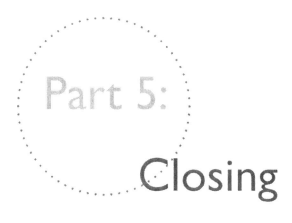

Part 5:

Closing

Use it or lose it, try new things, don't be afraid of success, and get off the sideline. I have talked at length about all of these issues, motivations and just plain thoughts. I want you to feel that energy; I want you to blast off like a rocket and be so happy you can't stand it.

I found this paraphrased version of Soren Kierkegaard's thoughts, a parable as close as possible to my feelings toward life, translated beautifully by Anthol Gill from the "Fringes of Freedom."

A certain flock of geese lived together in a barnyard with high walls around it. Because the corn was good and the barnyard was secure, these geese would never take a risk. One day a philosopher goose came among them. He was a very good philosopher, and every week they listened quietly and attentively to his learned discourses. "My fellow travelers on the way of life," he would say, "can you seriously imagine that this barnyard, with great, high walls around it, is all there is to existence?"

"I tell you, there is another and a greater world outside, a world of which we are only dimly aware. Our forefathers knew of this outside world. For did they not stretch their wings and fly across the trackless wastes of desert and ocean, of green valley and wooded hill? But alas, here we remain in this barnyard, our wings folded and tucked into our sides, as we are content to puddle in the mud, never lifting our eyes to the heavens, which should be our home."

The geese thought this was a very fine lecturing. "How poetical," they thought. "How profoundly existential. What a flawless summary of the mystery of existence." Often the philosopher spoke of the advantages of flight, calling on the geese to be what they were. After all, they had wings, he pointed out. What were wings for, but to fly with? Often he reflected on the beauty and the wonder of life outside the barnyard, and the freedom of the skies. And every week the geese were uplifted, inspired, moved by the philosopher's message. They hung on his every word. They devoted hours, weeks, months to a thoroughgoing analysis and critical evaluation of his doctrines. They produced learned treatises on the ethical and spiritual implications of flight. All this they did. But one thing they never did. They did not fly! For the corn was good and the barnyard secure.

Our time to fly is now; our windows of opportunities are open, the world is in need and all we have to do is recognize that every one of us has that specialness—every one!

Use it or lose it, and jump through the window; it's a beautiful world we live in!

Change your trajectory, by just one percent, and make a massive difference in your life. Believe me, this is just the first in a series of many books that will become the benchmark of "Boomers Rock". I look forward to hearing your stories, your changes, and your adventures. Because it is through our joint effort, sharing, loving and helping each other that we all improve our QOL!

Good luck, and thank you for reading my book!

Tom Matt, 2012
Holt, Michigan

About The Author

Tom Matt is a small town Michigan boy who grew up playing baseball and football, just an average American kid. Like so many, he never took his talents seriously. And, like so many, he took ordinary jobs that led him to Southern California in 1980 with the hope of finishing college. Unfortunately, bad habits gave way to damaging substance addictions. He married, had a daughter, but his lifestyle led to divorce and more change.

In his mid-thirties, Tom realized that he had a serious issue with alcohol and sought help to change his ways. He moved back to Michigan with his daughter and began to live the life he was meant to enjoy.

In 1999, sober and starting to build back his health, Tom reconnected with a high school sweetheart whom he married in 2001. Change begat change, and Tom enrolled at Michigan State University, earning both Bachelor and Masters degrees in Telecommunication Information Studies and Management.

Building on that success, and convinced that fitness leads to improved quality of life, Tom pursued a personal training certification with the National Academy of Sports Medicine. While completing that program, Tom competed in the Flint All Natural Body Building contest in Flint Michigan, in April of 2010 and, as a rookie competitor, placed 3rd in the Grand Master category, utilizing only whole foods and strength training.

In 2011, Tom became the host of "Boomers Rock" on FTNS.co and has since then interviewed dozens of experts in the field of fitness, nutrition, finance, and

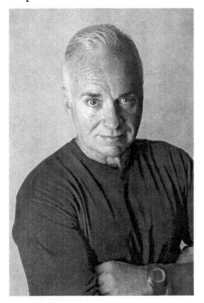

brain health. His personal mission is to help others improve the quality of their life. And who better to counsel those seeking help than someone who has made the mistake of venturing into the darkest tunnels life offers, but who found his way out and became a new man during the journey.

Bibliography

(Endnotes)

1   "Good to Great", Jim Collins, Harper Collins 2001

2   http://serendip.brynmawr.edu/Mind/Descartes.html

3   http://www.pbs.org/wgbh/aso/databank/entries/bhpenf.html

4   "You'll See It When You Believe It" by Wayne W. Dyer, Harper Publishing, 2001

5   "The Big Shift—Navigating the New Stage Beyond Midlife" by Marc Freedman, Public Affairs, 2011

6   http://en.wikipedia.org/wiki/Title_IX

7   http://www.wisegeek.com/what-is-neurogenesis.htm

8   http://en.wikipedia.org/wiki/Neuroglia

9   "The Brain That Changes Itself", Norman Doidge M.D. Viking Press, 2007

10 "The Secret Life of the Grown Up Brain", Barbara Strauch, Penguin Books 2010

11 "Adolescence" by Hall

12 "The Answer", John Assaraf and Murray Smith, Simon and Schuster 2008

13 "The Talent Code", Daniel Coyle, Bantom, 2009

14 "Outliers", Malcolm Gladwell, Little Brown and Company 2008

15 http://en.wikipedia.org/wiki/Big_Hairy_ Audacious_Goal

16 "Pizza Tiger" by Thomas Monaghan, Random House 1986

17 "Believe and Achieve" by Samuel Clement, Avon Books 1991

18 "The Power of Your Subconscious Mind", Joseph Murphy, Wilder/Public 2007

19 "Connected", ChrisTakis/Fowler, Little Brown 2009

20 http://www.earth.columbia.edu/sitefiles/file/ sachswriting/2012/worldhappinessreport.pdf

21   "Beyond the Relaxation Response" H. Benson with William Proctor, NY Times Books, 1984

22 http://www.unh.edu/health_services/ohep/ nutrition_non-diet.html

23 http://ontargetliving.com/

24 http://thewellnessrevolution.paulzanepilzer.com/ index.php

25 "Eating Well for Optimum Health", Andrew Weil M.D., Random House 2000

26 "Body for Life: 12 Weeks to Mental and Physical Strength" by Bill Phillips and Michael D'Orso (1999)

27 "Bad Science: Quacks, Hacks, and Big Pharma Flacks" by Ben Goldacre (Oct 2010)

28 http://www.sugar-and-sweetener-guide.com/ consumption-of-sugar.html

29 "The Omnivores Dilemma", Michael Pollan, Penguin Books 2006

30 "Eat, Drink and Be Healthy: The Harvard Medical School Guide to Healthy Eating" by Dr. Willett, Free Press 2005

31 "Fast Food Nation", Eric Schlosser, Houghton Mifflin 2004

32 http://www.rense.com/general12/wrong.htm

33 http://en.wikipedia.org/wiki/Baby_colic

34 www.webmd.com

35 "The Alzheimer's Action Plan", P. Murali Doraiswamy M.D., St. Martin's 2008

36 http://www.mayoclinic.org/news2012-sct/6700.html

37 "Spark" by Dr. John Ratey, Little, Brown 2008

38 http://www.scientificamerican.com/article.cfm?id=fitness-and-the-brain

39 http://www.alz.org/documents_custom/wad_press_release_2010.pdf

40 http://abcnews.go.com/US/wireStory?id=13462994#.TuDRz7I2GZQ

41 http://transgenerational.org/aging/demographics.htm#ixzz1fHStDqcy

42 http://www.michigan.org

43 "The Guru in You" by Yogi Cameron Alborzian, Harper One 2012

44 http://www.painmed.org/patient/facts.html#chronic

45 http://www.news-medical.net/news/2004/04/18/621.aspx

46 http://www.hippocratesinst.org/benefits-of-wheatgrass

47 http://www.organicfacts.net/organic-oils/organic-coconut-oil/health-benefits-of-coconut-oil.html

48 http://www.fishoilbenefit.net/fish-oil/carlson-fish-oil/n of the doctor.

49 http://juicing.mercola.com/sites/juicing/juicing.aspx

50 http://www.mayoclinic.com/health/flaxseed/AN01258

51 http://www.livestrong.com/article/30291-benefits-consuming-ground-flaxseed/#ixzz1dpI2wqcn

52 http://www.thehealthysnacksblog.com/2007/11/12/the-top-5-health-benefits-of-cinnamon/

53 http://bragg.com/

54 "Earl Mindell's Vitamin Bible" by Earl Mindell, Grand Central Life and Style 2011

55 "Healing With Whole Foods" by Paul Pitchford, North Atlantic Books, 2002

56 http://www.chlorellafactor.com/chlorella-spirulina-06.html

57 http://www.resveratrolbenefits.com/

58 http://www.wholeliving.com/134086/benefits-b-vitamins

59 http://www.mayoclinic.com/health/glucosamine/NS_patient-glucosamine

60 http://www.regenerativenutrition.com/boron-osteoporosis-arthritis-allergies-menopause-hormones.asp

61 http://tzpss.blogspot.com/2008/02/chondroitin-benefits-and-side-effects.html

62 http://www.green-tea-expert.com/green-tea-benefits.html

63 http://bragg.com/products/braggzyme-systemic-enzymes.html?gclid=CLrynvnFvawCFcvJKgodk DyDpg

64 http://www.preventive-health-guide.com/coq10.html

65 http://www.cnn.com/2009/HEALTH/11/04/aspirin.risk.heart.attacks/

66 http://vitamin-d-answers.info/

67 http://journals.lww.com/acsm-essr/abstract/2002/04000/exercise_enhances_and_protects_function.6.aspx

68 http://www.psychologytoday.com/basics/dopamine

69 http://www.livestrong.com/article/251785-exercise-and-its-effects-on-serotonin-dopamine-levels/#ixzz1fxYXsXqZ

70 http://www.angelfire.com/hi/TheSeer/seratonin.html

71 http://www.livestrong.com/article/202657-benefits-of-norepinephrine/#ixzz1gJnAAXKn

72 http://www.webmd.com/sleep-disorders/tc/melatonin-overview

CPSIA information can be obtained at www.ICGtesting.com
Printed in the USA
BVOW010549150113

310452BV00003BA/19/P